UROLOGIC CLINICS
OF NORTH AMERICA

Genitourinary Trauma

GUEST EDITOR
Jack W. McAninch, MD

CONSULTING EDITOR
Martin I. Resnick, MD

February 2006 • Volume 33 • Number 1

SAUNDERS

An Imprint of Elsevier, Inc.
PHILADELPHIA   LONDON   TORONTO   MONTREAL   SYDNEY   TOKYO

W.B. SAUNDERS COMPANY
A Division of Elsevier Inc.

1600 John F. Kennedy Boulevard • Suite 1800 • Philadelphia, Pennsylvania 19103-2899

http://www.theclinics.com

UROLOGIC CLINICS OF NORTH AMERICA	Volume 33, Number 1
February 2006	ISSN 0094-0143
Editor: Catherine Bewick	ISBN 1-4160-3562-1

Reprints. For copies of 100 or more, of articles in this publication, please contact the Commercial Reprints Department, Elsevier Inc., 360 Park Avenue South, New York, New York 10010-1710. Tel.: (212) 633-3813, Fax: (212) 462-1935, e-mail: reprints@elsevier.com.

The ideas and opinions expressed in *Urologic Clinics of North America* do not necessarily reflect those of the Publisher. The Publisher does not assume any responsibility for any injury and/or damage to persons or property arising out of or related to any use of the material contained in this periodical. The reader is advised to check the appropriate medical literature and the product information currently provided by the manufacturer of each drug to be administered to verify the dosage, the method and duration of administration, or contraindications. It is the responsibility of the treating physician or other health care professional, relying on independent experience and knowledge of the patient, to determine drug dosages and the best treatment for the patient. Mention of any product in this issue should not be construed as endorsement by the contributors, editors, or the Publisher of the product or manufacturers' claims.

Urologic Clinics of North America (ISSN 0094-0143) is published quarterly by W.B. Saunders, 360 Park Avenue South, New York, NY 10010-1710. Months of publication are February, May, August, and November. Business and Editorial Offices: 1600 John F. Kennedy Blvd., Suite 1800, Philadelphia, PA 19103-2899. Accounting and Circulation Offices: 6277 Sea Harbor Drive, Orlando, FL 32887-4800. Periodicals postage paid at New York, NY and additional mailing offices. Subscription prices are $210.00 per year (US individuals), $325.00 per year (US institutions), $240.00 per year (Canadian individuals), $390.00 per year (Canadian institutions), $280.00 per year (foreign individuals), and $390.00 per year (foreign institutions). Foreign air speed delivery is included in all *Clinics* subscription prices. All prices are subject to change without notice. **POSTMASTER:** Send address changes to *Urologic Clinics of North America*, Elsevier, Periodicals Customer Service, 6277 Sea Harbor Drive, Orlando, FL 32887-4800. **Customer Service: 1-800-654-2452 (US). From outside the US, call 1-407-345-4000.**

Urologic Clinics of North America is covered in *Index Medicus, Excerpta Medica, Current Contents/ Clinical Medicine, Science Citation Index,* and *ISI/BIOMED.*

Printed in the United States of America.

CONSULTING EDITOR

MARTIN I. RESNICK, MD, Lester Persky Professor and Chair, Department of Urology, School of Medicine, Case Western Reserve University, Cleveland, Ohio

GUEST EDITOR

JACK W. McANINCH, MD, Professor and Vice-Chair, Department of Urology, University of California School of Medicine, San Francisco; Chief of Urology, San Francisco General Hospital, San Francisco, California

CONTRIBUTORS

HOSAM S. AL-QUDAH, MD, Fellow of Trauma and Reconstructive Urology, Department of Urology, Wayne State University School of Medicine, Detroit, Michigan

NEJD F. ALSIKAFI, MD, Clinical Associate, Section of Urology, University of Chicago Pritzker School of Medicine; Department of Urology, Mount Sinai Medical Center, Chicago, Illinois

STEVEN BRANDES, MD, Associate Professor, Division of Urologic Surgery, Washington University School of Medicine, St. Louis, Missouri

JILL C. BUCKLEY, MD, Chief Resident, Department of Urology, University of California School of Medicine, San Francisco; Urology Service, San Francisco General Hospital, San Francisco, California

JOSEPH N. CORRIERE JR, MD, Professor of Urology, The University of Texas MD Anderson Cancer Center; Professor of Surgery (Urology), The University of Texas Medical School, Houston, Texas

SEAN P. ELLIOTT, MD, Clinical Instructor of Urology, Fellow in Traumatic and Reconstructive Urology, Department of Urology, University of California School of Medicine, San Francisco, San Francisco, California

EHAB A. ELTAHAWY, MD, Fellow, Adult and Pediatric Genitourinary Reconstructive Surgery, Eastern Virginia Medical School, Norfolk, Virginia

L. ANDREW EVANS, MD, Resident, Urology, Brooke Army Medical Center, Fort Sam Houston, Texas

GERALD H. JORDAN, MD, FACS, FAAP, Professor of Urology, Eastern Virginia Medical School, Norfolk; Director, Devine Center for Genitourinary Reconstructive Surgery, Sentara Norfolk General Hospital, Norfolk, Virginia

LAYRON LONG, MD, Resident, Department of Urology, University of Washington School of Medicine and Harborview Medical Center, Seattle, Washington

VIRAJ A. MASTER, MD, PhD, Assistant Professor of Urology, Emory University, Atlanta, Georgia

JACK W. McANINCH, MD, Professor and Vice-Chair, Department of Urology, University of California School of Medicine, San Francisco; Chief of Urology, San Francisco General Hospital, San Francisco, California

ALLEN F. MOREY, MD, Chief, Urology Service, Brooke Army Medical Center, Fort Sam Houston, Texas

DANIEL I. ROSENSTEIN, MD, FACS, FRCS (Urol), Associate Chief, Division of Urology, Santa Clara Valley Medical Center, San Jose; Clinical Instructor, Department of Urology, Stanford University Medical Center, Stanford, California

CARL M. SANDLER, MD, Professor of Radiology, The University of Texas MD Anderson Cancer Center and The University of Texas Medical School, Houston, Texas

RICHARD A. SANTUCCI, MD, Chief of Urology, Detroit Receiving Hospital; Associate Professor, Department of Urology, Wayne State University School of Medicine, Detroit, Michigan

RAMÓN VIRASORO, MD, Fellow, Adult and Pediatric Genitourinary Reconstructive Surgery, Eastern Virginia Medical School, Norfolk, Virginia

HUNTER WESSELLS, MD, FACS, Professor, Department of Urology, University of Washington School of Medicine; Chief of Urology, Harborview Medical Center, Seattle, Washington

CONTENTS

> Biosurgical preparations designed to promote surgical hemostasis and tissue adhesion are now available to the urologist and are increasingly being used across all surgical disciplines. Fibrin sealant and gelatin thrombin matrix are the two most widely used biosurgical adjuncts in urology. Complex reconstructive, oncologic, and laparoscopic genitourinary procedures are those most appropriate for sealant use. This article details the diverse urologic applications of biosurgical products in the management of urologic injuries and the promotion of wound healing.

> The kidney is the most commonly injured urologic organ and can sometimes be the most challenging to treat. Although most renal injuries may be treated successfully without operative intervention, it is important, and yet sometimes confusing, to delineate which cases should be managed with intervention and which may be observed. The common teaching that blunt renal injuries may be observed and penetrating injury must be explored may be true in most cases, but in select cases this dogma can be misleading and lead to poorer outcomes. The purpose of this article is to explain the important variables in the evaluation of renal trauma (clinical, radiologic, and sometimes surgical), how to stage renal trauma, and how to decide whether nonoperative or operative management is indicated.

> The decision to operate on a traumatized kidney should be made primarily on the basis of severity of injury to the kidney. Expanding or pulsatile retroperitoneal hematomas continue to be absolute indications for renal exploration. While parenchymal injuries, including severe parenchymal injuries, can usually be repaired, vascular injuries are generally less amenable to repair. Main renal arterial injuries should be repaired only if there

is a solitary kidney injury or a bilateral main renal artery injury. Such tools as the American Association for the Surgery of Trauma renal organ injury scale can help the urologist in managing injuries and in salvaging kidneys that would otherwise be removed.

these injuries are diagnosed, and explains classifications of urethral trauma. Timely and accurate diagnosis and classification of urethral injuries leads to appropriate acute management and reduced long-term morbidity.

Initial Management of Anterior and Posterior Urethral Injuries

Steven Brandes

The key to the initial management of a urethral injury is prompt diagnosis, accurate staging of the injury, and properly selecting an intervention that minimizes the overall chances for the debilitating complications of incontinence, impotence, and urethral stricture. Although somewhat controversial, blunt traumatic posterior injuries generally are managed best by primary realignment (when feasible), straddle injuries of the bulbar urethra by suprapubic urinary diversion, and penetrating urethral injuries by primary repair and urinary diversion.

Reconstruction and Management of Posterior Urethral and Straddle Injuries of the Urethra

Gerald H. Jordan, Ramón Virasoro, and Ehab A. Eltahawy

Urethral stricture disease, once associated mainly with gonococcal urethritis, is now most frequently a consequence of trauma, such as a fall-astride injury or a pelvic fracture. This article discusses issues and approaches related to the treatment of strictures associated with perineal straddle trauma and pelvic fracture urethral distraction defects. The authors emphasize that endoscopic procedures seldom cure these strictures and indwelling stents are seldom useful in treatment. Primary anastomotic techniques are associated with success rates in the high 90% range and appear to be remarkably durable in most cases. In contrast, tubed reconstruction of the urethra is inevitably associated with diminished success rates and with problems of durability.

Diagnosis and Management of Testicular Ruptures

Jill C. Buckley and Jack W. McAninch

Testicular ruptures are a common occurrence in scrotal trauma that can go undetected if a thorough examination or scrotal ultrasonography is not performed. Timely operative exploration and reconstruction is the standard of care and leads to high testicular salvage rates with hormonal, reproductive, and cosmetic benefits for the patient.

Penile and Genital Injuries

Hunter Wessells and Layron Long

Genital injuries are significant because of their association with injuries to major pelvic and vascular organs that result from both blunt and penetrating mechanisms, and the chronic disability resulting from penile, scrotal, and vaginal trauma. Because trauma is predominantly a disease of young persons, genital injuries may profoundly affect health-related quality of life and contribute to the burden of disease related to trauma. This article reviews the mechanism, initial evaluation, and operative management of injuries to the male and female external genitalia including the penis, scrotal skin, and vaginal structures.

Index

GOAL STATEMENT

The goal of *Urologic Clinics of North America* is to keep practicing urologists and urology residents up to date with current clinical practice in urology by providing timely articles reviewing the state of the art in patient care.

ACCREDITATION

The *Urologic Clinics of North America* is planned and implemented in accordance with the Essential Areas and Policies of the Accreditation Council for Continuing Medical Education (ACCME) through the joint sponsorship of the University of Virginia School of Medicine and Elsevier. The University of Virginia School of Medicine is accredited by the ACCME to provide continuing medical education for physicians.

The University of Virginia School of Medicine designates this educational activity for a maximum of 60 category 1 credits per year, 15 category 1 credits per issue, toward the AMA Physician's Recognition Award. Each physician should claim only those credits that he/she actually spent in the activity.

The American Medical Association has determined that physicians not licensed in the US who participate in this CME activity are eligible for AMA PRA category 1 credit.

Category 1 credit can be earned by reading the text material, taking the CME examination online at http://www.theclinics.com/home/cme, and completing the evaluation. After taking the test, you will be required to review any and all incorrect answers. Following completion of the test and evaluation, your credit will be awarded and you may print your certificate.

FACULTY DISCLOSURE/CONFLICT OF INTEREST

The University of Virginia School of Medicine, as an ACCME accredited provider, endorses and strives to comply with the Accreditation Council for Continuing Medical Education (ACCME) Standards of Commercial Support, Commonwealth of Virginia statutes, University of Virginia policies and procedures, and associated federal and private regulations and guidelines on the need for disclosure and monitoring of proprietary and financial interests that may affect the scientific integrity and balance of content delivered in continuing medical education activities under our auspices.

The University of Virginia School of Medicine requires that all CME activities accredited through this institution be developed independently and be scientifically rigorous, balanced and objective in the presentation/discussion of its content, theories and practices.

All authors/editors participating in an accredited CME activity are expected to disclose to the readers relevant financial relationships with commercial entities occurring within the past 12 months (such as grants or research support, employee, consultant, stock holder, member of speakers bureau, etc.). The University of Virginia School of Medicine will employ appropriate mechanisms to resolve potential conflicts of interest to maintain the standards of fair and balanced education to the reader. Questions about specific strategies can be directed to the Office of Continuing Medical Education, University of Virginia School of Medicine, Charlottesville, Virginia.

The authors/editors listed below have identified no professional or financial affiliations for themselves or their spouse/partner:
Hosam S. Al-Qudah, MD; Nejd F. Alsikafi, MD; Catherine Bewick, Acquisitions Editor; Steven B. Brandes, MD; Jill C. Buckley, MD; Joseph N. Corriere, Jr.; MD; Sean P. Elliot, MD; Ehab A. Eltahawy, MD; L. Andrew Evans, MD; Layron O. Long, MD; Viraj A. Master, MD, PhD; Jack W. McAninch, MD; Col. Allen F. Morey, MD, FACS; Martin Resnick, MD, Consulting Editor; Daniel I. Rosenstein, MD, RCS(C); Carl M. Sandler, MD; and, Ramon Virasoro, MD.

The authors/editors listed below identified the following professional or financial affiliations for themselves or their spouse/partner:
Gerald H. Jordan, MD is an employee and investigator for Engineers and Doctors – US Inc.
Richard A. Santucci, MD, FACS is on the speakers' bureau for Merck, Bayer, Boehringer, and Pfizer.
Hunter Wessells, MD is an independent contractor with Engineers and Doctors, and is on the Advisory Board for Palatin Technologies.

Disclosure of Discussion of non-FDA approved uses for pharmaceutical products and/or medical devices:
The University of Virginia School of Medicine, as an ACCME provider, requires that all faculty presenters identify and disclose any "off label" uses for pharmaceutical and medical device products. The University of Virginia School of Medicine recommends that each physician fully review all the available data on new products or procedures prior to instituting them with patients.

TO ENROLL

To enroll in the Urologic Clinics of North America Continuing Medical Education program, call customer service at 1-800-654-2452 or visit us online at www.theclinics.com/home/cme. The CME program is available to subscribers for an additional fee of $195.00

FORTHCOMING ISSUES

RECENT ISSUES

ELSEVIER
SAUNDERS

Urol Clin N Am 33 (2006) xi

UROLOGIC
CLINICS
of North America

Foreword

Genitourinary Trauma

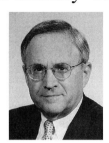

Martin I. Resnick, MD
Consulting Editor

Evaluation and management of patients who have traumatic injuries to the genitourinary tract have undergone significant changes over the past 2 decades. New approaches have been significantly influenced by the experience and observations of Dr. Jack McAninch, the guest editor of this issue of *Urologic Clinics of North America.* Not too long ago, surgical exploration of renal and urethral injuries was the norm, but with improvements in imaging techniques and the recognition that many patients can be successfully managed with observation alone, fewer and fewer patients who have these injuries are brought to the operating room. Renal injuries of significant magnitude that are associated with hemorrhage and urinary extravasation do surprisingly well with observation. Similarly, some patients with partial urethral injuries may not require immediate intervention and simple urethral catheter drainage may be all that is necessary. Finally, it has become recognized that not all bladder injuries require

exploration; with proper delineation of the injury, urethral catheter placement with appropriate observation may be the preferred approach. Surgical exploration is at times necessary for all of these injuries and the indications as well as the appropriate surgical techniques are well described by the various contributors to this monograph.

In this issue, Dr. McAninch and his colleagues address many of these approaches and the information presented will be of value to urologists, general surgeons, emergency physicians, and others caring for the traumatized patient.

Martin I. Resnick, MD
Department of Urology
School of Medicine
Case Western Reserve University
11100 Euclid Avenue
Cleveland, OH 44106

E-mail address: mir@po.cwru.edu

UROLOGIC
CLINICS
of North America

Urol Clin N Am 33 (2006) xiii

Preface
Genitourinary Trauma

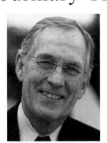

Jack W. McAninch, MD
Guest Editor

Traumatic injuries are the leading cause of death in young people in the United States. Indeed, in the past 3 years, gunshot injuries in the United States have resulted in as many deaths as were incurred by US forces during the entire Vietnam war. Clearly, traumatic injuries continue to be a major public health problem.

With the development of trauma centers and the specialty of trauma surgery, we continue to improve the care of the injured. A major member of the trauma team is the urologic surgeon, whose expertise in diagnosis and management of urologic and genital injuries results in reduced morbidity and mortality in trauma patients.

This issue of the *Urologic Clinics of North America* provides the reader with the most current information about the acute care and subsequent reconstruction of traumatic genitourinary system injuries. Since 1989 and the last issue on genitourinary trauma, new techniques and approaches have evolved for the treatment of many individual organ injuries. The use of hemostatic agents and tissue glues, as described by Dr. Morey, demonstrates the advances made to aid in organ salvage and reconstruction. Excellent imaging of urinary and genital injuries has facilitated accurate staging and increased non-operative management. Operative exploration, when indicated, can now result in high salvage rates.

All areas of genitourinary system injuries are addressed by a roster of distinguished authors, all leaders in the field, to bring detailed, practical, and up-to-date information on diagnosis and management of these traumatic injuries.

Jack W. McAninch, MD
Department of Urology
San Francisco General Hospital
1001 Potrero Avenue, Suite 3A210
San Francisco, CA 94110

E-mail address: jmcaninch@urol.ucsf.edu

ELSEVIER
SAUNDERS

Urol Clin N Am 33 (2006) 1–12

**UROLOGIC
CLINICS
of North America**

Hemostatic Agents and Tissue Glues in Urologic Injuries and Wound Healing

L. Andrew Evans, MD, Allen F. Morey, MD*

Urology Service, Brooke Army Medical Center, 3851 Roger Brooke Drive, Fort Sam Houston, TX, USA

Although most applications are off-label, tissue sealants and hemostatic agents are being used increasingly across all surgical disciplines. Biosurgical compounds can serve as adjuncts to primary surgical therapy or may assist in managing or preventing surgical complications. In urology, hemostatic agents and tissue sealants are finding increasing roles in managing traumatic and iatrogenic urologic injuries and promoting optimal wound healing

Among the variety of hemostatic products now available in the United States (Table 1), fibrin sealant and gelatin matrix thrombin are the most widely used biosurgical agents in urologic surgery. This article details the diverse urologic applications of these products for hemostasis, tissue adhesion, and urinary tract sealing.

Fibrin sealant

Development-

Mixtures of coagulation factors have been used in surgery for almost a century, dating back to the use of a fibrin emulsion by Bergel in 1909 to promote wound healing [1]. Purified thrombin became available in 1938 and was first combined with fibrinogen in 1944 to enhance adhesion of skin grafts to burned soldiers [2]. Although commercial fibrin sealant has been widely used in Europe since the 1970s, concerns about possible viral

transmission limited sealant use in the United States until recently. In 1998, Tisseel® (Baxter Health care, Deerfield, Illinois) became the first fibrin sealant approved by the Food and Drug Administration (FDA) for use in the United States.

Although the three FDA-approved indications for fibrin sealant are reoperative cardiac surgery, colon anastomosis, and treatment of splenic injury, fibrin sealants have been successfully used in countless numbers of nonurologic surgical applications, including liver laceration [3], hepatic resection [4], bowel and vascular anastomoses [5,6], enterocutaneous [7] and anorectal fistulae [8] closure, cardiothoracic surgery [9], neurosurgery [10], and embryo transfer [11]. A review in 2002 by Shekarriz and Stoller [12] was the first major contemporary urologic publication addressing the use of fibrin sealant in urologic surgery, and an increasing number of urologic sealant applications have followed.

Composition

Fibrin sealant contains two major components (thrombin and highly concentrated fibrinogen) that replicate and augment the final stage of the coagulation cascade—the cleavage of fibrinogen into fibrin by the action of thrombin—when mixed together. The fibrinogen concentration of sealant is supraphysiologic, 15 to 25 times higher than that of circulating plasma. The resultant clot tends to form more rapidly and more reliably than normal. Other key components of fibrin sealant are Factor XIII, which covalently crosslinks the fibrin polymer to produce an insoluble fibrin coagulum, and an antifibrinolytic agent which inhibits fibrinolysis thus preserving the stable fibrin clot (Fig. 1).

The views expressed in this article are those of the authors and do not reflect the official policy or position of the Department of Defense or other departments of the US Government.

* Corresponding author.

E-mail address: allen.morey@amedd.army.mil (A.F. Morey).

0094-0143/06/$ - see front matter. Published by Elsevier Inc.
doi:10.1016/j.ucl.2005.10.004

Table 1
Hemostatic agents and tissue adhesive available in the United States

Component	Brand Name	Manufacturer
Hemostatic Agents		
Fibrin sealant	Tisseel VH®	Baxter Healthcare
	Crosseal®	Omrix Biopharmaceuticals, Ltd
Gelatin Matrix thrombin sealant	FloSeal®	Baxter Healthcare
Thrombin	Thrombin-JMI®	Jones Pharma
Gelatin sponge	Gelfoam®	Pharmacia Upjohn
Oxidized cellulose	Surgicel®	Ethicon
Collagen sponge	Actifoam®	CR Bard
Collagen fleece	Avitene®	CR Bard
Recombinant Factor VIIa	NovoSeven®	Novo Nordisk A/S
Tissue Adhesives		
Fibrin sealant	Tisseel VH®	Baxter Healthcare
	Crosseal®	Omrix Biopharmaceuticals, Ltd
Polyethylene glycol	CoSeal®	Baxter Healthcare
Cyanoacrylate	Dermabond®	Ethicon

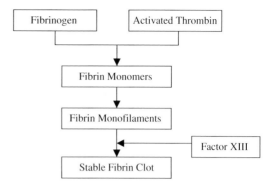

Fig. 1. Mechanism of action of liquid fibrin sealant in recapitulating the terminal portion of the coagulation cascade.

Tisseel® (Baxter Health care, Deerfield, Illinois) and Crosseal® (Omrix Biopharmaceuticals, Ltd, Israel) are the two fibrin sealants currently marketed in the United States. Tisseel contains bovine aprotinin as its antifibrinolytic agent. Aprotinin is a serine protease inhibitor derived from bovine lung that works to limit fibrinolysis by inhibiting plasmin, kallikrein, and trypsin. Crosseal uses only human-derived proteins by including tranexamic acid as its antifibrinolytic agent instead of bovine aprotinin. Tranexamic acid is a synthetic analog of the amino acid lysine and competes for lysine binding sites on plasminogen and plasmin, preventing binding to fibrin and inhibiting fibrinolysis [13].

Safety

All approved fibrin sealant preparations use a combination of donor screening, serum testing and retesting after 90 days storage, and a two-step vapor heating process to ensure viral safety [14,15]. These steps are highly effective in ensuring viral safety and, to our knowledge, in 2005, no transmissions of blood-borne viral pathogens associated with the use of FDA-approved fibrin sealants have yet been reported [14]. One

parvovirus B19 transmission involving a non-FDA approved fibrin sealant was reported from Japan, but most adults have preexisting antibodies to this virus and the infection is usually a self-limited diarrhea [16].

Delivery methods

Fibrin sealants are administered using a dual-chamber delivery system in which one chamber containing fibrinogen and factor XIII is admixed with the other chamber containing thrombin directly at the site of application using a "Y" adaptor, allowing an immediate conversion of fibrinogen to fibrin as the solutions exit the syringe [17]. Dual lumen catheters ensure smooth, rapid sealant delivery, and various specialized catheters and cannulae are available for endoscopic, laparoscopic, and open surgical application. A dual lumen peripherally inserted central catheter line for percutaneous transrenal application also has been used successfully [18]. Polymerization into the biocompatible fibrin clot is completed within 3 minutes [19], and the clot is broken down gradually and removed from the site by macrophages within 2 to 4 weeks, eventually becoming histopathologically invisible, without fibrosis or foreign-body reaction [20].

Urologic applications

Commercial fibrin sealant is used for three major reasons in urologic surgery—as a hemostatic agent, a urinary tract sealant, or a tissue adhesive. A list of the most common urologic applications is presented in Box 1. Fibrin sealant's unique properties as a hemostatic agent, urinary tract sealant, and tissue adhesive make it an

---

Box 1. Urologic applications of fibrin sealant

I. Hemostasis
Partial nephrectomy
　Open [21,22]
　Laparoscopic [23–26]
Percutaneous nephrolithotomy [27]
Management of splenic injury [28]
Hemophilia and other coagulopathy
　[29–31]
Circumcision [30,31]
Hemorrhagic cystitis [32]

II. Urinary tract sealant
Laparoscopic and open pyeloplasty
　[33–46]
Ureteral anastomoses [33–36]
Urethral reconstruction [37]
Simple retropubic prostatectomy [38]
Radical retropubic prostatectomy [39]
Vasovasostomy and
　vasoepididymostomy [40–42]
Bladder injury [29]
Lymphadenectomy [43,44]
Percutaneous nephrolithotomy tract
　closure [27]

III. Tissue adhesion
Fournier's gangrene reconstruction
　[45,46]
Fistula closure [29,47,48]
Skin grafting [46]
Orchiopexy [49,50]
Penile chordee [51]
Complex urethroplasty [37]

---

effective adjunct for managing complex urologic injury and promoting wound healing in the genitourinary tract.

Hemostasis

Partial nephrectomy

Fibrin sealant has been used since 1979 in open partial nephrectomy [21,52]. The recent advent of minimally invasive techniques for nephron sparing surgery has resulted in widespread fibrin sealant use during laparoscopic partial nephrectomy today [22–25]. A recent survey of 193 members of the World Congress of Endourology discovered 68% of surgeons routinely used fibrin sealant to assist with hemostasis during laparoscopic partial nephrectomy [26]. Application of fibrin sealant to the cut surface of the renal parenchymal wound after segmental vascular and collecting system suture ligation during partial nephrectomy enhances hemostasis. The fibrin sealant layer can then be supported by a gelatin or collagen bolster, which is glued effectively into the renal defect by holding manual pressure on the bolster "sandwich." In vivo testing of fibrin sealant in a porcine model of open partial nephrectomy demonstrated supraphysiologic sealing pressures of the renal parenchymal vasculature (mean 378 mm Hg) and collecting system (mean 166 mm Hg) compared with unsealed controls [53].

Renal trauma

In 1989, Kram and colleagues first reported fibrin sealant use in 14 patients who presented with traumatic renal injuries; renal salvage was achieved always with no postoperative infection, delayed hemorrhage, or urinoma formation [54]. In 2004, the authors' laboratory reported the effective use of FDA-approved fibrin sealant in central porcine renal stab wounds when used in conjunction with a bolster of absorbable gelatin sponge or microfibrillar collagen [55]. Though not yet available commercially, the absorbable fibrin adhesive bandage, a similar product consisting of dry fibrin sealant on a polyglactin mesh backing developed in conjunction with the American Red Cross, significantly reduced bleeding in addition to operative and ischemic times in repair of porcine models of lower renal pole amputation [56] and Grade IV renal stab wounds [57].

Miscellaneous hemostatic applications

Noller and colleagues reported no hemorrhagic complications in 10 consecutive renal units treated with fibrin sealant-assisted tubeless percutaneous nephrolithotomy (PCNL) [27]. The instillation of 2 to 3 mL of fibrin sealant into the parenchymal defect is performed as the sheath is removed at the conclusion of PCNL in lieu of nephrostomy drainage. Postoperative computed tomography (CT) imaging has confirmed the absence of perirenal hematomas in these "tubeless" procedures.

Intraoperative splenic injury during left nephrectomy is managed easily with direct application of fibrin sealant to the bleeding parenchyma, thereby promoting prompt hemostasis and avoiding the need for splenectomy [28]. Fibrin sealant also has been used successfully to control "medical" bleeding caused by warfarin use or other coagulopathies during urologic surgical procedures [29–31]. Other urologic hemostatic applications include sealing the oral mucosal donor site during buccal graft urethroplasty [58] and cystoscopic application of fibrin sealant after fulguration to provide hemostasis in refractory radiation-induced hemorrhagic cystitis after supravesical urinary diversion [32].

Urinary tract sealant

Various nonurologic studies have suggested the increased strength of sealed anastomoses. Skin sutures supported by a layer of fibrin sealant provided watertight anastomoses immediately after surgery and withstood significantly higher hydrostatic pressures than nonsealed anastomoses [59]. Han and colleagues noted that microvascular sutured anastomoses supported by fibrin sealant had enhanced re-endotheliazation [59,60,61], and Park and colleagues reported significantly increased tensile strength in sealed skin closure versus controls [42].

Ureteral anastomosis

Kram and colleagues first reported the successful use of fibrin sealant as a bolster over the suture line for ureteral anastomosis in 1989 [54]. The authors have found fibrin sealant to be a useful adjunct in managing various ureteral injuries, iatrogenic and traumatic, and frequently have performed "drain-free" sealed repairs. Between 2001 and 2003, 10 patients underwent definitive management of ureteral injury at the authors' institution. The authors' experience has shown that sealant effectively prevents ureteral urinary extravasation and has not been associated with postoperative infection, leak, or scar formation (Fig. 2). The authors' believe that a sealed, stented ureteral repair is prudent in cases where a transabdominal approach has been performed because transabdominal drains are avoided. The authors also believe the sealant should be applied as a means of "suture support" by reinforcing standard suture lines, not in lieu of careful suture repair.

The increasing performance of laparoscopic renal reconstruction surgery may lead to increased sealant use. Fibrin sealant has been shown to support approximating sutures successfully in a porcine model of laparoscopic ureteral anastomoses [33] and has improved radiographic outcomes compared with free needle suturing and laser weld closure [34]. Various studies have shown fibrin sealant to be effective as a bolster for laparoscopic pyeloplasty or collecting system repair [35], and satisfactory drainage has been confirmed by radiologic imaging at 1 to 2 years [36].

Prostatectomy

Drain-free, simple, retropubic prostatectomy has been performed successfully in over 25 cases in the authors' institution, and a faster return to regular diet and shortened hospital stay when compared with conventional simple prostatectomy have been demonstrated [38]. Again, the sealant should be applied outside the urinary tract, over the sutured prostatic capsular closure, to ensure that the fibrin clot does not occlude urinary catheter drainage. Similarly, Diner and colleagues

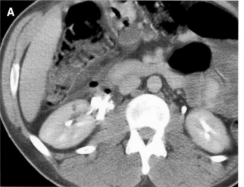 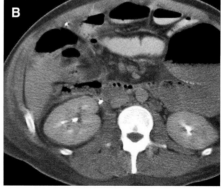

Fig. 2. (*A*) Stab wound to right flank with medial perirenal contrast extravasation on preoperative trauma computed tomography (CT). A 4-cm laceration to the right renal pelvis successfully repaired using 5-zero PDS suture with the application of a bolster of 5 mL of fibrin sealant over the suture line to reinforce urinary tract seal. No drain was placed. (*B*) Postoperative CT image obtained 72 hours later demonstrates drain-free intact repair over ureteral stent without evidence of extravasation or urinoma.

reported in 2004 that a significant decrease in postoperative drain output was noted in 16 patients following radical retropubic prostatectomy when 5 mL of fibrin sealant was applied to the suture line of the urethrovesical anastomosis [39]. Earlier drain removal should facilitate a more expedient recovery and earlier discharge from the hospital leading to cost savings.

Urethroplasty

Fibrin sealant seems to allow earlier catheter removal, improved patient satisfaction, and enhanced wound healing after pendulous urethroplasty [37]. In our experience of applying fibrin sealant directly over a suture line of 5-zero polydiaxanone during pendulous urethroplasty in 18 patients, a completely healed anastomosis was confirmed by voiding cystourethrography performed 1 week postoperatively in 83% of patients; all 18 patients demonstrated complete healing within 14 days compared with 8% of patients in the control group who had persistent extravasation at 21 days postoperatively ($P < .05$). Pendulous urethral reconstruction seems to be uniquely well-suited for sealant use because the superficial nature of the urethra in this location does not provide the robust surrounding spongy tissues that are found routinely in the bulbar urethra (Fig. 3).

Complication management

Fibrin sealant seems to promote the successful transvaginal management of iatrogenic cystotomy sustained during transvaginal hysterectomy. The authors observed that direct transvaginal fibrin sealant injection functions well as a bolster interposition over the cystotomy repair thus preventing the additional time and morbidity required for abdominal bladder repair or tissue

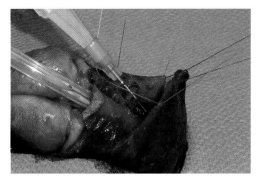

Fig. 3. Application of fibrin sealant as a bolster over the suture line of pendulous urethroplasty.

interposition with a Martius or omental flap [29]. Fibrin sealant also has been used to prevent lymphocele formation after lymphadenectomy [43]. Used as a sclerosant after percutaneous drainage of postoperative lymphoceles in renal transplantation, instillation of fibrin sealant achieved complete resolution of the lymphocele in 75% of patients without the need for open surgical management [44]. Percutaneous transrenal application of 5 mL of fibrin sealant across a refractory calyceal urinary leak secondary to gunshot wound has proven effective in sealing refractory collecting system injury [18].

Tissue adhesion

Tissue planes

The fibrin polymer resulting from fibrin sealant application facilitates wound healing by increasing tissue plane adherence thus eliminating dead space, accelerating revascularization, reducing hemorrhage, preventing seroma, and minimizing inflammation [62,63].

Tissue sealant properties of fibrin sealant have been applied to reduce air leaks and bronchopleural fistulae after pulmonary resection and decortication [64,65], secure skin grafts in reconstructive and burn surgery [66], and occlude chronic enterocutaneous [7] and anorectal [8] fistulous tracts.

Fibrin sealant now is used routinely at the authors' institution during complex urethroplasty, especially cases requiring panurethral reconstruction (Fig. 4). The scrotum is bivalved completely to provide wide access to the underlying diseased urethra, and the scrotal wings are glued together with sealant after urethral repair to prevent edema and hematoma. Similar efficacy has been reported in 17 patients undergoing complex genital reconstructive surgery, such as spit-thickness skin grafting and thigh flap surgery for Fournier's gangrene sequelae and invasive penile cancer: 94% of patients recovered without infection, seroma, hematoma, or other complications (Fig. 5) [45,46].

Urinary tract fistulae

In addition to sealing tissue planes, fibrin sealant promotes closure of urinary fistulae by promoting the local proliferation of fibroblasts and subsequent replacement by connective tissue, allowing for occlusion of the fistulous tract [15]. The fibrin polymer promotes the ingrowth of fibroblasts during wound healing and an influx of immune cells is stimulated in a paracrine fashion [67]. The complex interaction of neutrophils, macrophages, and fibroblasts provides the basis of

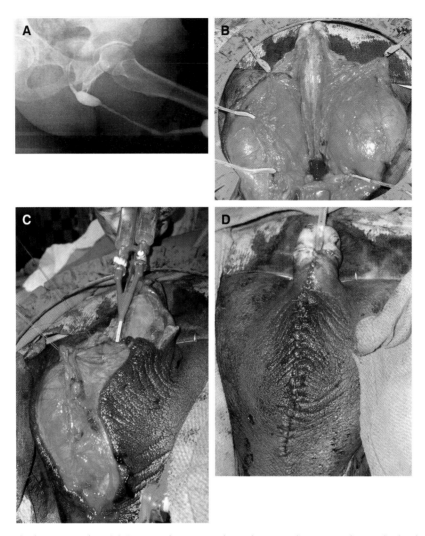

Fig. 4. Panurethral reconstruction. (*A*) Preoperative retrograde urethrogram shows extensive urethral stricture. (*B*) Penile base, scrotum, and perineum are bivalved completely, thus allowing excellent exposure for urethral reconstruction. Buccal grafts were required in this case to reconstruct a 17-cm defect. Fibrin sealant is applied as a bolster to the suture lines and as a tissue adhesive to glue the scrotal wings back together with good hemostasis. (*C*) Application of fibrin selant to glue scrotal wings together after urethral reconstruction. (*D*) Postoperative result after scrotum is glued and sutured back together shows no ecchymosis, edema, or drain requirement.

wound contraction and remodeling necessary for healthy wound healing. The recent application of the Vacuum Assisted Closure® (VAC®, Kinetic Concepts, Inc., San Antonio, Texas) device in closing larger complex wounds is believed to function through similar cellular mechanisms [68].

Morita and Tokue reported the successful closure of a radiation-induced vesicovaginal fistula with the endoscopic injection of fibrin sealant in combination with bovine collagen [47]. Three serial injections of fibrin sealant allowed for complete continence in the case of a ureterocutaneous fistula following cadaveric kidney transplantation [48]. The authors reported the definitive treatment of six cases of vesicocutaneous and urethrocutaneous fistulae by sealing the tract with the direct injection of 5 mL commercial fibrin sealant after endoscopic fulguration with 100% success [29] (Fig. 6). The authors have not found sealant to be effective in vesicovaginal fistula, however, and this is probably because these fistulas are too short and broad compared with the long, thin fistulas

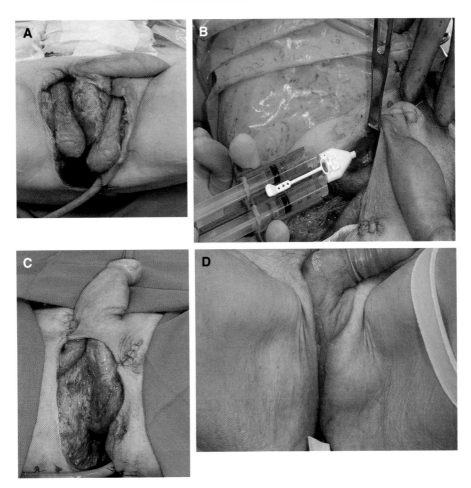

Fig. 5. Successful Fournier's gangrene reconstruction assisted by fibrin sealant. (*A*) Genital wound after initial debridement for perirectal necrotizing infection with extensive scrotal involvement. (*B*) Lateral view of same patient showing application of aerosolized fibrin sealant sprayed under local tissue flaps to enhance adherence, hemostasis, and promote wound healing. (*C*) Final appearance immediately after secondary debridement shows surrounding skin flaps mobilized to shrink the tissue defect, glued into place with fibrin sealant. Catheter is in presacral cavity in area where necrotic rectum had previously been. (*D*) Final appearance after wound vac assisted closure 2 months postoperatively. No grafts or additional skin flaps were used to provide skin coverage. Testes are still buried in thigh pouches.

typically found extending from the lower urinary tract in males.

Other tissue glue applications

Fibrin sealant has been applied to urologic surgery as a tissue glue in several other areas, including vasovasostomy [40,41] and vasoepididymostomy [42]. Patency rates have been reported to be comparable to standard microsurgical technique but only limited clinical data in humans are available to date. Fibrin sealant has been used in orchiopexy after spermatic cord torsion. In an effort to reduce the known severe

inflammatory reaction induced by transparenchymal sutures in the tunica albuginea [69], Sencan demonstrated less inflammation and better preservation of seminiferous tubular diameter with the use of fibrin sealant for testis fixation in prepubertal rats [49]. Noeske previously reported adequate testicular fixation after placing fibrin sealant into the scrotal space followed by 5 minutes of manual compression [50]. Hafez and colleagues successfully used fibrin sealant to patch tunical defects created along the ventral aspect of the corpora cavernosa in a rabbit model to simulate the sutureless correction of penile chordee. Histologic examination at

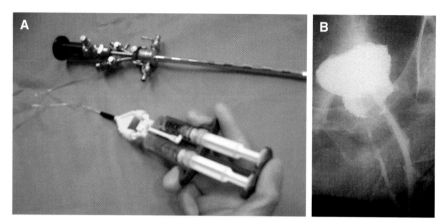

Fig. 6. (*A*) Cystoscopic injection by way of dual lumen catheter with "Y" adapter is one of several available devices for application of fibrin sealant. (*B*) In this case, sealant was delivered cystoscopically to close a urethrocutaneous fistula after endoscopic fulguration.

6 and 12 weeks showed regeneration of the tunica albuginea without evidence of residual fibrin sealant. Cavernosography failed to detect leakage of contrast from the site of previous fibrin sealant application [51].

Gelatin matrix thrombin

FloSeal® gelatin matrix thrombin solution (Baxter Health Care, Deerfield, Illinois), approved by the FDA in 1999, consists of a bovine-derived gelatin matrix of granules that are mixed with bovine thrombin solution before application. Since FloSeal® contains no fibrinogen, contact with blood is required for thrombin to convert endogenous fibrinogen to fibrin. As blood percolates through the matrix in the presence of bleeding, the granules swell approximately 20% within 10 minutes upon contact with blood, conforming to the shape of the wound and forming fibrin polymer [70]. Gelatin matrix is used best as a pure hemostatic agent not a tissue glue or urinary tract sealant.

Gelatin matrix thrombin solution now is used extensively to obtain hemostasis in open and laparoscopic nephron sparing surgery, even more so than fibrin sealant [71,72]. A recent survey revealed that 75% of laparoscopic urologic surgeons reported using FloSeal® as a hemostatic adjunct for laparoscopic partial nephrectomy (Fig. 7) [26]. Gill and colleagues found improved hemostasis (median blood loss 109 mL versus 200 mL) and decreased overall complication rates during laparoscopic partial nephrectomy when

FloSeal was applied to the partial nephrectomy bed before suture renorrhaphy was performed over a Surgicel© (Ethicon, Somerville, New Jersey) bolster [73]. Gelatin matrix thrombin also has been used to allow tubeless PCNL as previously described for fibrin sealant with favorable results [74].

FloSeal® seems to have a possible role in treatment of major traumatic renal injuries. In our laboratory, the authors have observed that application of FloSeal® to complex porcine renal injuries produced significantly less mean blood loss and time to hemostasis independent of whether primary renal arterial occlusion was performed [75]. Again, further laboratory study is required to substantiate the possible urinary tract sealant properties of gelatin matrix.

Safety considerations

Fibrin sealant should not be placed into large blood vessels because of the risk for potential thromboembolism, although this has not been clinically reported. The use of bovine-derived proteins carries a risk for allergic reaction upon re-exposure to the material, although bovine aprotinin (found in fibrin sealant) is much less immunogenic than thrombin [76–79].

Repeat use of bovine thrombin preparations, which also contain bovine factor V, can induce the formation of antibodies that cross-react with human factor V and lead to a coagulopathic state [80]. Pavlovich reported the postoperative development of coagulopathy caused by repeat exposure to bovine thrombin during partial nephrectomy [81].

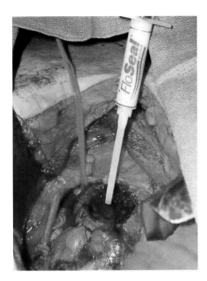

Fig. 7. Application of FloSeal® to renal parenchymal wound after partial nephrectomy has been shown to reduce complications.

The reported incidence of hypersensitivity to intravenous thrombin approaches 10%; therefore, fibrin sealant containing bovine protein products should be used with caution in patients previously exposed to aprotinin [82].

Future considerations

Recombinant factor VIIa

Approved by the FDA for the treatment of hemophiliacs with factor VIII and IX deficiency, recombinant factor VIIa (rFVIIa) (NovoSeven®; Novo Nordisk A/S, Denmark) is a powerful systemic hemostatic agent which has been used successfully off-label to obtain hemostasis in critically ill patients who present with severe coagulopathy as a result of impaired liver function or trauma [83]. The landmark study demonstrating rFVIIa, could reduce blood loss and transfusion requirements in patients who present with a normal native coagulation system originated in urologic surgery. The first randomized placebo-controlled trial of this agent by Friederich and colleagues studied the effect of administering rFVIIa (20 or 40 mcg/kg) or placebo at the beginning of retropubic prostatectomy. Recombinant factor VIIa (40 mcg/kg) resulted in a 50% reduction of blood loss compared with placebo and eliminated the need for blood transfusion, which was required in approximately 60% of patients in the placebo arm [84]. Further study is required to better elucidate optimal dosing and to define which urologic

surgical applications may best benefit from this powerful new agent. Presently, cost considerations of factor VIIa remain prohibitive for routine use.

Summary

Hemostatic agents and tissue sealants should not be viewed as a replacement for sound surgical judgment or technique but rather as complementary adjuncts to improve surgical outcome. Fibrin sealant offers an effective adjunct for hemostasis, reinforcement of urinary tract seal, and adhesion of tissue planes. Numerous reports in virtually all surgical disciplines have confirmed the reliable enhancement of wound healing promoted by fibrin sealant. Gelatin matrix thrombin solution provides exceptional hemostatic properties for complex surgical wounds, such as partial nephrectomy. Future development of novel biotherapeutic materials continue to provide urologists with safe, reliable agents for managing challenging urogenital injuries and complications.

References

[1] Bergel S. Uber Wirkungen des Fibrins. Dtschr Med Wochenschr 1909;35:633–65.

[2] Cronkite EP, Lozner EL, Deaver J. Use of thrombin and fibrinogen in skin grafting. JAMA 1944;124: 976–8.

[3] Cohn SM, Cross JH, Ivy ME, et al. Fibrin glue terminates massive bleeding after complex hepatic injury. J Trauma 1998;45:666–72.

[4] Wakasugi J, Shimada H. Application of fibrin sealant in liver surgery. Biomedical Progress 1994;7: 75–80.

[5] Kjaergard HK. Suture support: is it advantageous. Am J Surg 2001;182:15S–20S.

[6] Milne A, Murphy W, Reading S, et al. A randomized trial of fibrin sealant in peripheral vascular surgery. Vox Sang 1996;70:210–2.

[7] Hwang TL, Chen MF. Short note: randomized trial of fibrin tissue glue for low output enterocutaneous fistula. Br J Surg 1996;83:112.

[8] Park JJ, Cintron JR, Orsay CP, et al. Repair of chronic anorectal fistulae using commercial fibrin sealant. Arch Surg 2000;135:166–9.

[9] Rousou J, Levitsky S, Gonzalez-Lavin L, et al. Randomized clinical trial of fibrin sealant in patients undergoing resternotomy or reoperation after cardiac operations. A multicenter study. J Thorac Cardiol Surg 1989;97:194–203.

[10] Sawamura Y, Asaoka K, Terasaka S, et al. Evaluation of application techniques of fibrin sealant to prevent cerebrospinal fluid leakage: a new device

for the application of aerosolized fibrin glue. Neurosurgery 1999;44:332–7.

[11] Ben-Rafael Z, Ashkenazi J, Shelef M, et al. The use of fibrin sealant in in vitro fertilization and embryo transfer. Int J Fertil Menopausal Stud 1995;40: 303–6.

[12] Shekarriz B, Stoller ML. The use of fibrin sealant in urology. J Urol 2002;167:1218–25.

[13] Dunn CJ, Goa KL. Tranexamic acid: a review of its use in surgery and other indications. Drugs 1999;57: 1005–32.

[14] Jackson MR. Fibrin sealants in surgical practice: an overview. Am J Surg 2001;182:S1–7.

[15] Spotnitz WD. Commercial fibrin sealants in surgical care. Am J Surg 2001;182:8S–14S.

[16] Hino M, Ishiko O, Honda KI, et al. Transmission of symptomatic parvovirus B19 infection by fibrin sealant used during surgery. Br J Haematol 2000;108: 194–5.

[17] Wozniak G. Fibrin sealants in supporting surgical techniques: the importance of individual components. Cardiovas Surg 2003;11(Suppl 1):17–21.

[18] Baughman SM, Morey AF, Van Geertruyden PH, et al. Percutaneous transrenal application of fibrin sealant for refractory urinary leak after gunshot wound. J Urol 2003;170:522–3.

[19] Sapala JA, Wood MH, Schuhknecht MP. Anastomotic leak prophylaxis using a vapor heated fibrin sealant: report on 738 gastric bypass patients. Obes Surg 2004;14:35–42.

[20] Martinowitz U, Saltz R. Fibrin sealant. Curr Opin Hematol 1996;3:395–402.

[21] Levinson AK, Swanson DA, Johnson DE, et al. Fibrin glue for partial nephrectomy. Urology 1991;38: 314–6.

[22] Wolf J, Seifman B, Montie J. Nephron sparing surgery for suspected malignancy: open surgery compared to laparoscopy with selective use of hand assistance. J Urol 2000;163:1659–64.

[23] Janetschek G, Daffner P, Peschel R, et al. Laparoscopic nephron sparing surgery for small renal cell carcinoma. J Urol 1998;159:1152–5.

[24] Pruthi RS, Chun J, Richman M. The use of a fibrin tissue sealant during laparoscopic partial nephrectomy. BJU Int 2004;93:813–7.

[25] Finley DS, Lee DI, Eichel L, et al. Fibrin glue-oxidized cellulose sandwich for laparoscopic wedge resection of small renal lesions. J Urol 2005;173: 1477–81.

[26] Gerber GS, Stockton BR. Trends in endourologic practice. Laparoscopic partial nephrectomy. J Endourol 2005;19:21–4.

[27] Noller MW, Baughman SM, Morey AF, et al. Fibrin sealant enable tubeless percutaneous stone surgery. J Urol 2004;172:166–9.

[28] Canby-Hagino ED, Morey AF, Jatoi I, et al. Fibrin sealant treatment of splenic injury during open and laparoscopic nephrectomy. J Urol 2000; 164:2004–5.

[29] Evans LA, Ferguson KH, Foley JP, et al. Fibrin sealant for the management of genitourinary injuries, fistulas and surgical complications. J Urol 2003;169:1360–2.

[30] Martinowitz U, Varon D, Jonas P, et al. Circumcision in hemophilia: the use of fibrin glue for local hemostasis. J Urol 1992;148:855–7.

[31] Avanoglu A, Celik A, Ulman I, et al. Safer circumcision in patients with hemophilia: the use of fibrin glue for local hemostasis. BJU Int 1999;83:91–4.

[32] Ouwenga MK, Langston MD, Campbell SC. Use of fibrin sealant in recalcitrant hemorrhagic cystitis. J Urol 2004;172:1348.

[33] McKay TC, Albala DM, Gehrin BE, et al. Laparoscopic ureteral anastomosis using fibrin glue. J Urol 1994;152:1637–40.

[34] Wolf JS Jr, Soble JJ, Nakada SY, et al. Comparison of fibrin glue, laser weld, and mechanical suturing device for the laparoscopic closure of ureterotomy in a porcine model. J Urol 1997;157:1487–92.

[35] Patel R, Caruso RP, Taneja S, et al. Use of fibrin glue and gelfoam to repair collecting system injuries in a porcine model: implications for the technique of laparoscopic partial nephrectomy. J Endourol 2003; 17:799–804.

[36] Eden CG, Sultana SR, Murray KH, et al. Extraperitoneal laparoscopic dismembered fibrin-sealant pyeloplasty: medium-term results. Br J Urol 1997; 80:382–9.

[37] Hick EJ, Morey AF. Initial experience with fibrin sealant in pendulous urethral reconstruction. Is early catheter removal possible? J Urol 2004;171:1547–9.

[38] Morey AF, McDonough RC, Kizer WS, et al. Drain-free simple retropubic prostatectomy with fibrin sealant. J Urol 2002;168:627–9.

[39] Diner EK, Patel SV, Kwart AM. Does fibrin sealant decrease immediate urinary leakage following radical retropubic prostatectomy? J Urol 2005;173: 1147–9.

[40] Silverstein JI, Mellinger BC. Fibrin sealant vasal anastomosis compared to conventional sutured vasovasostomy in the rat. J Urol 1991;145:1288–91.

[41] Vankemmel O, Rigot JM, Burnouf T, et al. Delayed vassal reanastomosis in rats: comparison of a microsurgical technique and a fibrin-glue procedure. BJU Int 1996;78:271–4.

[42] Shekarriz BM, Thomas AJ Jr, Sabanegh E, et al. Fibrin-glue assisted vasoepididymostomy: a comparison to standard end-to-side microsurgical vasoepididymostomy in the rat model. J Urol 1997;158: 1602–5.

[43] Janetschek G, Hobisch A, Hittmar A, et al. Laparoscopic retroperitoneal lymphadenectomy after chemotherapy for stage IIB nonseminomatous testicular carcinoma. J Urol 1999;161:477–81.

[44] Chin AI, Ragavendra N, Hilborne L, et al. Fibrin sealant sclerotherapy for treatment of lymphoceles following renal transplantation. J Urol 2003;170: 380–3.

[45] Decastro BJ, Morey AF. Fibrin sealant for the reconstruction of fournier's gangrene sequelae. J Urol 2002;167:1774–6.

[46] Morris MS, Larson RJ, Santucci RA, et al. Role of fibrin sealant as tissue glue in complex genital reconstructive surgery. J Urol 2004;171S:19.

[47] Morita T, Tokue A. Successful endoscopic closure of radiation induced vesicovaginal fistula with fibrin glue and bovine collagen. J Urol 1999;162:1689.

[48] Tsurusaki T, Sakai H, Nishikido M, et al. Occlusion therapy for an intractable transplant-ureteral fistula using fibrin glue. J Urol 1996;155:1698.

[49] Sencan A, Genc A, Gunsar C, et al. Testis fixation in prepubertal rats: fibrin glue versus transparenchymal sutures reduces testicular damage. Eur J Pediatr Surg 2004;14:193–7.

[50] Noeske M. The use of fibrin sealant adhesive alone after torsion of the spermatic cord. Fibrin sealing in surgical and nonsurgical fields: gynecology and obstetrics. Urology. In: Schlag DW, Melchior H, editors. Heidelberg (DEU): Springer-Verlag; 1994. p. 91.

[51] Hafez AT, El-Assmy A, El-Hamid MA. Fibrin glue for the suture-less correction of penile chordee: a pilot study in a rabbit model. BJU Int 2004;94:433–6.

[52] Urlesberger H, Rauchenwald K, Henning K. Fibrin adhesives in surgery of the renal parenchyma. Eur Urol 1979;5:260–1.

[53] Kouba E, Tornehl C, Lavelle J, et al. Partial nephrectomy with fibrin glue repair: measurement of vascular and pelvicaliceal hydrodynamic bond integrity in a live and abbatoir porcine model. J Urol 2004;172:326–30.

[54] Kram HB, Ocampo HP, Yamaguchi MP, et al. Fibrin glue in renal and ureteral trauma. Urology 1989;33:215–8.

[55] Griffith BC, Morey AF, Rozanski TA, et al. Central renal stab wounds: treatment with augmented fibrin sealant in a porcine model. J Urol 2004;171: 445–7.

[56] Cornum RL, Morey AF, Harris R. Does the absorbable fibrin adhesive bandage facilitate partial nephrectomy? J Urol 2000;164:864–7.

[57] Morey AF, Anema JG, Harris R, et al. Treatment of grade 4 renal stab wounds with absorbale fibrin adhesive bandage in a porcine model. J Urol 2001;165: 955–8.

[58] Riccabona M. Reconstruction or substitution of the pediatric urethra with buccal mucosa: indications, technical aspects and results. Tech Urol 1999;5: 133–8.

[59] Oosterlinck W, Cheng H, Hoebeke P, et al. Watertight sutures with fibrin glue: an experimental study. Eur Urol 1993;23:481–4.

[60] Han SK, Kim SW, Kim WK. Microvascular anastomosis with minimal suture and fibrin glue: experimental and clinical study. Microsurgery 1998;18: 306–11.

[61] Park W, Kim WH, Lee CH, et al. Comparison of two fibrin glues in anastomoses and skin closure. J Vet Med A Physiol Pathol Clin Med 2002;49: 385–9.

[62] Spotnitz WD, Falstrom JK, Rodeheaver GT. The role of sutures and fibrin sealant in wound healing. Surg Clin North Am 1997;77:651–69.

[63] Bold EL, Wanamaker JR, Zins JE, et al. The use of fibrin glue in the healing of skin flaps. Am J Otolaryngol 1996;17:27–30.

[64] Mouritzen C, Dromer M, Keinecke HO. The effect of fibrin glueing to seal bronchial and alveolar leakages after pulmonary resections and decortications. Eur J Cardiothorac Surg 1993;7:75–80.

[65] York EL, Lewall DB, Hirji M, et al. Endoscopic diagnosis and treatment of postoperative bronchopleural fistula. Chest 1990;97:1390–2.

[66] Greenhalgh DG, Gamelli RL, Lee M, et al. Multicenter trial to evaluate the safety and potential efficacy of pooled human fibrin sealant for the treatment of burn wounds. J Trauma Inj Infect Crit Care 1999; 46:433–40.

[67] Gorodetsky R, Vexler A, An J, et al. Haptotactic and growth stimulatory effects of fibrin(ogen) and thrombin on cultured fibroblasts. J Lab Clin Med 1998;131:269–80.

[68] Whelan C, Stewart J, Schwartz BF. Mechanics of wound healing and importance of vacuum assisted closure in urology. J Urol 2005;173:1463–70.

[69] Dixon TK, Ritchey ML, Boykin W, et al. Transparenchymal suture fixation and testicular histology in a prepubertal rat model. J Urol 1993;149:1116–8.

[70] Summary of safety and effectiveness. FloSeal matrix hemostatic sealant. United States Food and Drug Administration; 2000. PMA P990009.

[71] Richter F, Schnorr D, Deger S, et al. Improvement of hemostasis in open and laparoscopically performed partial nephrectomy using a gelatin matrix-thrombin tissue sealant (Floseal). Urology 2003;61: 73–7.

[72] User HM, Nadler RB. Applications of FloSeal in nephron-sparing surgery. Urology 2003;62:342–3.

[73] Gill IS, Ramani AP, Spaliviero M, et al. Improved hemostasis during laparoscopic partial nephrectomy using gelatin matrix thrombin sealant. Urology 2005;65:463–6.

[74] Lee DI, Uribe C, Eichel L, et al. Sealing percutaneous nephrolithotomy tracts with gelatin matrix hemostatic sealant: initial clinical use. J Urol 2004; 171:575–8.

[75] Hick EJ, Morey AF, Harris RA, et al. Gelatin matrix treatment of complex renal injuries in a porcine model. J Urol 2005;173:1801–4.

[76] Beierlein W, Scheule AM, Antoniadis G, et al. An immediate, allergic skin reaction to aprotinin after reexposure to fibrin sealant. Transfusion 2000;40:302–5.

[77] Cohen DM, Norberto J, Cartabuke R, et al. Severe anaphylactic reaction after primary exposure to aprotinin. Ann Thorac Surg 1999;67:837–8.

[78] Scheule AM, Beierlein W, Lorenz H, et al. Repeated anaphylactic reactions to aprotinin in fibrin sealant. Gastrointest Endosc 1998;48: 83–5.

[79] Fastenau DR, McIntyre JA. Immunochemical analysis of polyspecific antibodies in patients exposed to bovine fibrin sealant. Ann Thorac Surg 2000;69: 1867–72.

[80] Christie RJ, Carrington L, Alving B. Postoperative bleeding induced by topical bovine thrombin: report of two cases. Surgery 1997;121:708–10.

[81] Pavlovich CP, Battiwalla M, Rick ME, et al. Antibody induced coagulopathy from bovine thrombin use during partial nephrectomy. J Urol 2001;165: 1617.

[82] MacGillivray TE. Fibrin sealants and glues. J Card Surg 2003;18:480–4.

[83] Khan AZ, Parry JM, Crowley WF, et al. Recombinant factor VIIa for the treatment of severe postoperative and traumatic hemorrhage. Am J Surg 2005; 189:331–4.

[84] Friederich PW, Henny CP, Messelink EJ, et al. Effect of recombinant activated factor VII on perioperative blood loss in patients undergoing retropubic prostatectomy: a double-blind placebo-controlled randomized trial. Lancet 2003;361:201–5.

ELSEVIER
SAUNDERS

Urol Clin N Am 33 (2006) 13–19

UROLOGIC
CLINICS
of North America

Staging, Evaluation, and Nonoperative Management of Renal Injuries

Nejd F. Alsikafi, MD[a,b,*],
Daniel I. Rosenstein, MD, FACS, FRCS (Urol)[c,d]

[a]Department of Urology, Mount Sinai Medical Center, 1500 South California Avenue, F934, Chicago, IL, 60608, USA
[b]Section of Urology, University of Chicago Pritzker School of Medicine, Chicago, IL, USA
[c]Division of Urology, Santa Clara Valley Medical Center, San Jose, CA, USA
[d]Department of Urology, Stanford University Medical Center, Stanford, CA, USA

The kidney is the most commonly injured urologic organ and may be the most challenging to treat. Although most renal injuries may be treated successfully without operative intervention, it is important and yet sometimes confusing to delineate which cases should be managed with intervention and which may be observed. The common teaching that blunt renal injuries may be observed and penetrating injury must be explored may be true in most cases, but in select cases this dogma can be misleading and lead to poorer outcomes. The purpose of this article is to explain the important variables in the evaluation of renal trauma (clinical, radiologic, and surgical), how to stage renal trauma, and how to decide whether nonoperative or operative management is indicated.

Evaluation

When the trauma patient enters the trauma bay, a thorough evaluation and treatment protocol ensues led by the emergency department (ED) physician or the surgical trauma team. The purpose of these maneuvers is to collect and assess clinical information and the likelihood of traumatic injuries. An assessment of clinical history, physical examination findings and radiologic findings all help form the presumptive diagnoses and treatment plan. The focus of this section relies exclusively on the evaluation of renal trauma.

Clinical history

The mechanism of injury is helpful in determining likelihood of traumatic injuries. A distinction should be made for blunt versus penetrating trauma. For blunt injuries a history of rapid deceleration (eg, motor vehicle accident or fall from heights) or a direct blow to the flank are important indicators of potential renal trauma. For penetrating trauma, location of entrance and exit wounds may help determine the likelihood of renal injury. Additionally, the type of firearm and the caliber and velocity of the bullet (high versus low) are important determinants of blast injury. In stab wounds, the length of the knife should be ascertained as it would help determine the likelihood and degree of penetration into the kidney or other abdominal organs.

In many of these injuries concomitant abdominal injuries are likely and must be evaluated. In penetrating injuries, nearly all patients with renal gunshot wounds and up to 60% of patients with renal stab wounds have injury to adjacent organs [1–3]. The management of other abdominal injuries affects appropriate management of the renal injury.

Clinical evaluation

In adult renal trauma especially, the two most important indicators for significant injury are hematuria, defined as less than five cells per high power field (HPF) as seen from the first aliquot of

---

* Corresponding author. Department of Urology, Mount Sinai Medical Center, 1500 South California Avenue, F934, Chicago, IL, 60608.
E-mail address: nalsikafi@yahoo.com (N.F. Alsikafi).

urine of a catheterized specimen, and hypotension, defined as a systolic blood pressure less than 90 mm/Hg at anytime before resuscitation. The first aliquot of urine is important and intravenous (IV) resuscitation dilutes the urine. Additional indicators for possible renal injury include the presence of a flank hematoma, abdominal or flank tenderness, rib fractures, and penetrating injuries to the low thorax or flank.

Hematuria is important as it may represent significant urologic injury. In most cases, a low correlation exists between severity of renal injury and degree of hematuria [4–6]; however, in cases of an isolated flank injury (especially in isolated penetrating trauma), the presence of any degree of hematuria carries a significant risk for renal parenchymal injury. Additionally, hypotension is important as it may signify significant hemorrhage from the renal parenchyma or renal pedicle. Hematuria is absent frequently in renal pedicle injuries. Interestingly, hematuria is not seen in up to 36% of renal pedicle injuries and in 24% of renal artery occlusions [7,8].

Hematuria and hypotension also are important variables in determining which renal trauma patients need to undergo radiologic imaging. In a large study from San Francisco General Hospital, no significant renal injuries were missed in adult blunt renal trauma patients without gross hematuria, hypotension, or significant mechanism (rapid deceleration, high falls) [9]. This study concluded that these select patients safely may avoid imaging for staging purposes. These patients often have minor renal injuries that may be treated with observation. In the rare patient who sustains

a significant renal injury, concomitant abdominal injuries always occur that necessitate radiologic evaluation for staging. In those with gross hematuria or microscopic hematuria and shock, a higher incidence of significant renal injuries exists, necessitating imaging for staging purposes (Fig. 1).

Radiographic evaluation

The criteria for radiologic imaging include 1) all penetrating trauma patients with a likelihood of renal injury (abdomen, flank, or low chest) who are hemodynamically stable, 2) all blunt trauma with significant mechanism of injury, specifically rapid deceleration as would occur in a motor vehicle accident or a fall from heights, 3) all blunt trauma with gross hematuria, 4) all blunt trauma with hypotension defined as a systolic pressure of less than 90 mm/Hg, and 5) all pediatric patients with greater 5 red blood cell (RBC)/HPF [10]. Patients who are hemodynamically unstable after initial resuscitation require surgical intervention. Delaying definitive therapy to obtain a preoperative imaging study in an unstable patient is not warranted and may compromise resuscitative efforts.

Computerized tomography

The single best radiologic modality for diagnosing renal injury is computerized tomography (CT) [5,11]. CT is rapid, is widely-available in trauma centers, gives excellent three-dimensional data, and accurately can diagnose urinary extravasation, renal contusions, depth of renal lacerations, nonviable tissue, and renal pedicle injuries

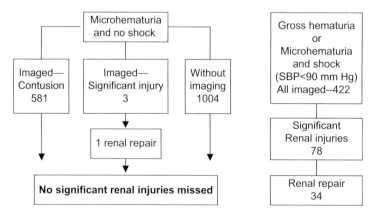

Fig. 1. Algorithm demonstrating that in adults who present with blunt trauma, imaging studies may be performed selectively. (*From* Miller KS, McAninch JW. Radiographic assessment of renal trauma: our 15-year experience. J Urol 1995;154:352–5; with permission.)

[12,13]. CT's ability to provide anatomic and functional data when used with IV contrast is useful in staging renal injuries. Additionally, CT is useful in diagnosing concomitant abdominal injuries.

Because of the increased use of rapid spiral CT scans, an adequate renal assessment cannot be made without delayed images. On the first set of images, IV contrast does not have enough time to fill the collecting system and, as a result, urinary extravasation and collecting system injuries may be missed. A second series of delayed films must be obtained 5 to 10 minutes after the initial IV bolus of contrast to visualize adequately most parenchymal and collecting system injuries with acceptable accuracy.

Findings on CT scan that suggest major injury include (1) medial hematoma, especially with extravasation on the early phase implying renal vascular injury; (2) medial extravasation on the delayed films suggesting renal pelvic injury or disruption of the proximal ureter; and (3) any lack of parenchymal contrast on the early phase suggesting arterial injury (Table 1).

Intravenous pyelogram

Formerly the most commonly used modality for imaging renal trauma was the IV pyelogram (IVP). It was proved to be less effective in diagnosing significant renal injury than CT. In one study, urinary extravasation and nonfunction are seen in less than 50% of patients with major or vascular injuries [14,15]. In another study, 82% of patients who sustain significant renal injury had an indeterminate IVP, whereas CT provided a definitive diagnosis in all patients [16]. Additionally, IVP is time-consuming and labor-intensive and only visualizes the urinary tract. In short, CT has a higher sensitivity and specificity in the evaluation of blunt renal trauma as compared with IVP and is the imaging modality of choice [16,17]. A limited role exists for intraoperative

Table 1
CT findings suggestive of major injury

CT findings	Major injury
Medial hematoma	Renal pedicle injury
Medial extravasation	Renal pelvic injury or ureteropelvic junction disruption
Lack of parenchymal contrast	Arterial injury

IVP in the surgical staging of an unstable patient, which is discussed later.

MRI

MRI equals CT in correctly grading blunt renal injuries and particularly in detecting the presence and size of perirenal hematomas. An advantage of MRI is its ability to differentiate old hematoma from a more recent hematoma by differences in signal intensity. Although MRI can replace CT in patients with iodine allergy and may be helpful in patients with equivocal findings on CT, it should be reserved for selected patients because of increased cost and increased imaging time [18].

Angiography

In penetrating injuries, angiography is the second study of choice behind CT because reliably it can stage significant injury and offers the possibility of embolization. In a stable patient who presents with persistent bleeding, angiography may allow selective arterial embolization, which may obviate the need for surgical exploration [19].

Ultrasound

Although ultrasonography has gained popularity in the rapid diagnosis of intraabdominal injuries in the trauma setting, its efficacy in diagnosis of renal trauma is lacking. Several studies have documented its inferiority, including one study in which 78% of known renal injuries were read as negative [20]. Despite being quick, available, transportable, and inexpensive, ultrasonography is agreed upon not to be the modality of choice.

Surgical evaluation

Surgical staging of renal injuries is performed in patients who are too unstable to undergo a complete clinical or radiologic evaluation. These patients have often undergone life-threatening injuries and are rushed to the operating room for definitive treatment before adequate radiologic assessment may be performed. In these cases, after the patient is explored and stabilized by the trauma surgeon, an effort to stage the renal injury is performed. In these cases a one-shot IVP is performed 10 minutes after IV infusion of 2 mg/kg of contrast material. The main purpose of the one-shot intraoperative IVP is to assess the presence of a functioning contralateral kidney and to radiographically stage the injured side. The one-shot IVP may also be used in the setting of an unexpected retroperitoneal hematoma and may help to determine if the kidneys are injured and how well they function. In a recent review [21], a normal intraoperative one-shot IVP obviated the need for renal exploration.

If the IVP findings are not normal, renal exploration should be performed and the injuries assessed. Before opening the retroperitoneal space early vascular control should be considered. The need for early vascular control is debatable as some studies conclude that it is a time-consuming maneuver with no change in nephrectomy rate [22], while others claim benefit [23]. After the kidney is exposed on all sides and is examined, if the injury is significant and the patient is stable, renorrhaphy should be performed. If the patient is unstable, the injury is irreparable, or the injury would simply take too much time to repair in a time-critical situation, nephrectomy should be considered.

Staging

The most widely accepted classification used to stage renal trauma was developed by the American Association for Surgery of Trauma (AAST) Organ Injury Scaling Committee. It stages renal injuries with five different grades, shown in Table 2 and Fig. 2.

Grade I is classified as a renal contusion or a small, nonexpanding, subcapsular hematoma. Grade II is defined as a renal laceration confined to the cortex of the kidney (<1 cm) without urinary extravasation or a nonexpanding perirenal hematoma. Grade III injuries are lacerations which extend into the medulla (>1 cm) without evidence of urinary extravasation. Grades IV and V each have a parenchymal and a vascular component. In Grade IV injuries, the parenchymal injury extends through the cortex and medulla into the collecting system with evidence of urinary extravasation, whereas the vascular component includes a main renal arterial or venous thrombosis or injury with a contained hematoma. Grade V parenchymal injuries include a shattered kidney, indicating multiple Grade IV lacerations, whereas the vascular component includes complete pedicle avulsion. No mention is made in the classification for segmental vascular injuries.

The AAST kidney injury scale has been validated by several studies. In the largest study, an analysis of greater than 2500 renal injuries from a single institution was reviewed retrospectively and showed that the scale correlates with the need for kidney repair or removal [24].

Table 2

American Association for the Surgery of Trauma Organ Injury Severity Scale for the Kidney (from Moore EE, Shackford SR, Pachter HL, et al. Organ injury scaling; Spleen, liver, and kidney. J Trauma 1989; 29: 1664–1666)

Grade	Type	Description
I	Contusion	Microscopic or gross hematuria, urologic studies normal
	Hematoma	Subcapsular, nonexpanding without parenchymal laceration
II	Hematoma	Nonexpanding perirenal hematomoa confined to renal retroperitoneum
	Laceration	<1 cm parenchymal depth of renal cortex without urinary extravasation
III	Laceration	>1 cm parenchymal depth of renal cortex without urinary extravasation
IV	Laceration	Parenchymal laceration extending through renal cortex, medulla, and collecting system
	Vascular	Main renal artery or vein injury without contained hemorrhage
V	Laceration	Completely shattered kidney
	Vascular	Avulsion of the renal hilum, devascularizing the kidney

Data from Moore EE, Shackford SR, Pachter HL, et al. Organ injury scaling; Spleen, liver, and kidney. J Trauma 1989;29:1664–66.

Nonoperative management

In determining whether a renal injury needs to be explored several factors must be considered. These factors include (1) the presence of concomitant injuries and their management, (2) the presence of continued hemodynamic instability after initial resuscitation, and (3) the stage and mechanism of the renal injury (Fig. 3).

From a practical point of view, the management of concomitant injuries often dictate the ultimate approach used to treat renal injuries. If a patient is going to the operating room for associated abdominal injures or profound instability, the urologist should be present. After initial stabilization and exploration is complete, at the

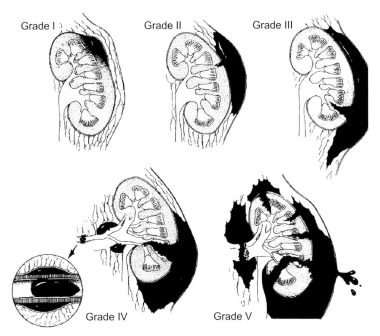

Fig. 2. The American Association for Surgery of Trauma renal injury scale. (*From* Moore EE, Shackford SR, Pachter HL, et al. Organ injury scaling; spleen, liver, and kidney. J Trauma 1989;29:1664–6; with permission.)

discretion of the trauma surgeon, the urologist should stage the renal injury adequately (if it has not been done preoperatively) with a one-shot intraoperative IVP or with operative exploration. Based on these findings, the urologist determines whether the kidney must be explored, repaired, or observed. Exploration should ensue in settings of an expanding or pulsatile retroperitoneal hematoma or no visualization of injured the kidney on the one-shot IVP. Exploration should be considered in settings of incomplete staging, urinary extravasation outside of Gerota's fascia, or

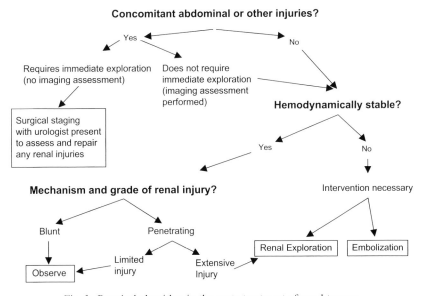

Fig. 3. Practical algorithm in the acute treatment of renal trauma.

devitalized tissue especially in the setting of pancreatic injury or fecal spillage as higher rates of postoperative infected urinomas and perinephric abscesses are more common [25]. In times when hemodynamic instability is ongoing and the source of the blood loss is from the kidney or its pedicle, nephrectomy may be necessary. In the hands of urologists clearly nephrectomy more often is performed because of irreparable injury rather than the patient's hemodynamic instability [26].

In patients who have less severe or no other abdominal injuries after evaluation from the trauma surgeon and do not go for immediate abdominal exploration, the presence hemodynamic instability and the degree and mechanism of the renal injury guides the urologists' management. Hemodynamic instability in these cases often is from the kidney, and bleeding, hematoma, urinary extravasation, and devascularized tissue should be ascertained from postinjury imaging. In situations of mild hemodynamic instability and parenchymal injury after a penetrating injury, such as in an isolated renal stab wound, renal angiography with embolization may be a viable treatment option [27]. In cases of more extensive injury, operative exploration of the kidney may be necessary.

In hemodynamically stable patients with penetrating injuries who are completely staged, select patient cohorts may be treated nonoperatively. Limited renal injuries are more suitable for this approach. In one study [28], Grade II injuries fared well when treated nonoperatively. In this study, some Grade III and IV injuries also were managed nonoperatively. Although most resolved uneventfully, delayed renal bleeding occurred in 23.5% of these patients. Some of these delayed bleeds may have been amenable to angioembolization afterward.

In patients with blunt trauma, most injuries initially may be managed nonoperatively. Even in settings of urinary extravasation and nonviable tissue bluntly injured kidneys seem to heal well when managed conservatively. In a series of over 2900 blunt renal injuries from San Francisco General Hospital renal trauma database, only 2.6% of patients were managed operatively with less than a 0.7% nephrectomy rate [26]. In most cases, urinary extravasation resolves without consequence, and in those that do not, placement of a ureteral stent or a percutaneous nephrostomy tube may be necessary for resolution, especially in injuries which involve the renal pelvis.

Renal injuries with nonviable segments also may be managed conservatively, though the complication rate and need for delayed surgical intervention is higher. One study suggests that there is an increase in patient morbidity in those with nonperfused renal segments versus those without in terms length of hospital stay, need for blood transfusions, and need for delayed surgical intervention [29]. In this study, six patients (30%) ultimately needed an open procedure for an infected urinoma, a perinephric abscess, or a delayed bleed. Another study, which examined the effect of nonviable renal segment between 25% and 50%, showed that nonoperative management yielded only a 6% nephrectomy rate, though 85% of patients sustained urologic complications amenable to salvage endourologic or percutaneous procedures. These complications included persistent urine leaks, infected urinoma, and perinephric abscesses [25].

Even Grade V shattered but perfused kidneys in hemodynamically stable, bluntly injured patients also have been treated successfully without surgery. In a series of six shattered but perfused kidneys, four (66%) kidneys functioned before discharge as determined by CT scan, and none of these patients subsequently developed hypertension though patient follow-up was poor [30].

Postinjury, all patients who are managed nonoperatively are placed on bed rest until their gross hematuria resolves. Additionally, all patients who present with urinary extravasation or nonviable tissue are imaged periodically while as an inpatient to monitor for injury resolution. Follow-up imaging also is performed to document renal function 3 months following injury.

Summary

With the proper evaluation of information obtained clinically, radiographically, or surgically, renal injuries can be staged adequately. In the clinically stable patients, an infused CT scan with delayed images provides ample data regarding the extent and severity of renal injury. In hemodynamically unstable patients, operative staging may be necessary and findings from the one-shot intraoperative IVP may be useful. Following the principles and algorithm described above, nonoperative management is employed most commonly in blunt renal injuries and may be used selectively in patients who present with penetrating injuries and a low likelihood of secondary complications, surgery, or renal loss.

References

[1] Sagalowski AI, McConnell JD, Peters PC. Renal trauma requiring surgery: an Analysis of 185 cases. J Trauma 1983;23:128–31.

[2] Jackson GL, Thal ER. Management of stab wounds of the back and flank. J Trauma 1979;19:660–4.

[3] Bernath AS, Schutte H, Fernandez RRD, et al. Stab wounds of the kidney: conservative management in flank penetration. J Urol 1983;129:468–70.

[4] Boone TB, Gilling PJ, Husmann DA. Ureteroplevic junction disruption following blunt abdominal trauma. J Urol 1993;150:33–6.

[5] Federle MP, Brown TR, McAninch JW. Penetrating renal trauma: CT evaluation. J Comp Assist Tomog 1987;11:1026–30.

[6] Palmer LS, Rosenbaum RR, Gershbaum MD, et al. Penetrating ureteral trauma at an urban trauma center: 10-year experience. Urology 1999;54:34–6.

[7] Cass AS. Renovascular injuries for external trauma. Urol Clin North Am 1989;16:213–20.

[8] Wilson RF, Ziegler DW. Diagnostic and treatment problems in renal injuries. Am Surg 1987;53:399–402.

[9] Miller KS, McAninch JW. Radiographic assessment of renal trauma: our 15-year experience. J Urol 1995;154:352–5.

[10] Buckley JC, McAninch JW. Pediatric renal injuries: management guidelines from a 25-year experience. J Urol 2004;172(2):687–90.

[11] Bretan PN Jr, McAninch JW, Federle MP, et al. Computerized tomographic staging of renal trauma: 85 consecutive cases. J Urol 1986;136:561–5.

[12] Carroll PR, McAninch JW, Klosterman P, et al. Renovascular trauma; risk assessment, surgical management, and outcome. J Trauma 1990;30:547–54.

[13] Lang EK. Arteriography in the assessment of renal trauma. The impact of arteriographic diagnosis on preservation of renal function and parenchyma. J Trauma 1975;15:553–66.

[14] Cass AS, Luxenberg M. Accuracy of computed tomography in diagnosing renal artery injuries. Urology 1989;34:249–51.

[15] Nicolaisen GS, McAninch JW, Marshall GA, et al. Renal trauma; re-evaluation of the indications for radiographic assessment. J Urol 1985;133:183–7.

[16] Cass AS, Viera J. Comparison of IVP and CT findings in patients with severe renal injury. Urology 1987;29(5):484–7.

[17] Halsell RD, Vines FS, Shatney CH, et al. The reliability of excretory urography as a screening examination for blunt renal trauma. Ann Emerg Med 1987;16:1236–9.

[18] Ku JH, Jeon YS, Kim ME, et al. Is there a role for magnetic resonance imaging in renal trauma? Int J Urol 2001;8:261–7.

[19] Uflacker R, Paolini RM, Lima S. Management of traumatic hematuria by selective renal artery embolization. J Urol 1984;132:662–7.

[20] McGahan JP, Richards JF, Jones CD, et al. Use of ultrasonography in the patient with acute renal trauma. J Ultrasound Med 1999;18:207–15.

[21] Morey AF, McAninch JW, Tiller BK, et al. Single shot intraoperative excretory urography for the immediate evaluation of renal trauma. J Urol 1999;161(4):1088–92.

[22] Golzalez RP, Falimirski M, Holevar MR, et al. Surgical management of renal trauma: is vascular control necessary? J Trauma 1999;47(6):1039–42.

[23] McAninch JW, Carroll PR. Renal trauma: kidney preservation through improved vascular control—a refined approach. J Trauma 1983;22:285–90.

[24] Santucci RA, McAninch JW, Safir M, et al. Validation of the American Association for the Surgery of Trauma organ injury severity scale for the kidney. J Trauma 2001;50(2):195–200.

[25] Hussman DA, Gilling PJ, Perry MO, et al. Major renal lacerations with devitalized fragment following blunt abdominal trauma: a comparison between nonoperative (expectant) versus surgical management. J Urol 1993;150(6):1774–7.

[26] Master VA, Young J, McAninch JW. Nephrectomy for traumatic renal injury: 26-year experience at San Francisco General Hospital. J Urol 2005;173(4):126A.

[27] Eastham JA, Wilson TG, Ahlering TE. Urologic evaluation and managment of renal proximity stab wounds. J Urol 1993;150(6):1771–3.

[28] Wessells H, McAninch JW, Meyer A, et al. Criteria for nonoperative treatment of significant penetrating renal lacerations. J Urol 1997;157(1):24–7.

[29] Moudouni SM, Patard JJ, Manunta A, et al. A conservative approach to major renal lacerations with urinary extravasation and devitalized renal segments. BJU Int 2001;87:290–4.

[30] Altman AL, Hass C, Dinchman KH, et al. Selective nonoperative management of blunt grade 5 renal injury. J Urol 2000;164:27–30.

ELSEVIER
SAUNDERS

Urol Clin N Am 33 (2006) 21–31

UROLOGIC
CLINICS
of North America

Operative Management of Renal Injuries: Parenchymal and Vascular

Viraj A. Master, MD, PhD[a], Jack W. McAninch, MD[b],*

[a]Department of Urology, Emory University, 1365 Clifton Road, Building B, Atlanta, GA 30322, USA
[b]Department of Urology, University of California, San Francisco, San Francisco General Hospital,
1001 Potrero Avenue, Suite 3A20 San Francisco, CA 94110, USA

Of all genitourinary organs, the kidney is the most likely to be injured in cases of external trauma and injuries to at least one kidney occur in as many as 10% of abdominal trauma cases. Today, most of these injuries can be managed by the urologist without requiring an operation thanks to advances in staging techniques resulting from increased use of CT scanning, as well as increased awareness, based on outcomes research, of the kidney's capacity for healing. Nonetheless, in certain cases, severely injured kidneys are best managed by exploration and reconstruction, with nephrectomy reserved for life-threatening hemorrhage or for kidneys that have been injured beyond repair. Ultimately, the objective of managing patients with severe kidney injuries is to prevent significant hemorrhage and retain enough functioning nephron mass to avoid end-stage kidney failure. A secondary goal is to avoid complications specifically attributable to the traumatized kidney.

The task of repairing an injured kidney begins with staging and evaluation. See the article by Alsikafi and Rosenstein elsewhere in this volume for further information about staging and evaluation. Also, note the algorithms for the management of penetrating renal trauma (Fig. 1) and blunt renal trauma (Fig. 2). Clinical staging begins with history and physical examination, including the determination of whether the patient has been in shock and whether hematuria is present.

Selective imaging, consisting of a CT scan, including delayed views at 5 to 10 minutes after the administration of intravenous contrast, should be performed if time permits to evaluate ureteral and renal pelvis injuries. The American Association for the Surgery of Trauma (AAST) has created a renal organ injury scale that correlates with patient outcomes, thus serving as a guide for appropriate and selective management (Table 1). This renal injury scale is one of the few classification schemes that has been prospectively validated and found to correlate directly with need for surgical intervention [1]. Grade 1 injuries include subcapsular hematomas and renal contusions (Fig. 3). Grade 2 injuries involve small lacerations into the renal cortex. Grade 3 injuries extend through the corticomedullary junction. Grade 4 injuries consist of injuries into the collecting system; or renal vascular injuries, such as main renal artery or vein injury with contained hemorrhage; or segmental vessel injury. Grade 5 injuries are life-threatening injuries and include kidneys with pedicle avulsion off the great vessels, as well as completely shattered kidneys.

Indications for surgical exploration

Most renal injuries are contusions or minor lacerations (AAST Grade 1 or 2 injuries), and may thus be managed nonoperatively if adequately staged. Appropriate radiographic staging has also permitted selective nonoperative management of major lacerations in both blunt and penetrating trauma (see Figs. 1 and 2 for management algorithms). In a recent series of Grade 4 lacerations at San Francisco General Hospital,

* Corresponding author.
E-mail address: jmcaninch@urol.ucsf.edu
(J.W. McAninch).

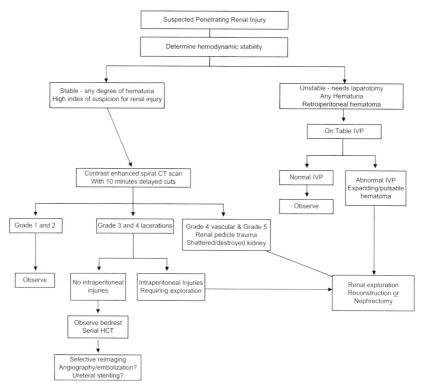

Fig. 1. Management algorithms for penetrating renal injury. (*Adapted from* Santucci RA, Wessells H, Bartsch G, et al. Evaluation and management of renal injuries: consensus statement of the Renal Trauma Subcommittee. BJU Int 2004;93:937.)

22% were successfully managed nonoperatively [2]. Penetrating injuries more commonly require laparotomy because of associated injuries or hemodynamic instability. In the San Francisco General Hospital experience, however, 55% of stab wounds and 24% of gunshot wounds were successfully managed expectantly through careful selection and complete clinical and radiographic staging [3]. If expectant management is selected in the setting of a major renal laceration, close monitoring with serial hematocrit measurements and liberal use of repeat imaging, especially at 36 to 48 hours, is indicated.

The absolute indications for surgical exploration in renal trauma are persistent, life-threatening hemorrhage believed to be from renal injury, renal pedicle avulsion, and expanding, pulsatile, or uncontained retroperitoneal hematoma. Patients with such injuries often present in severe shock. Thus, rarely have these patients undergone radiographic staging before emergency laparotomy [4]. In the setting of renal pedicle avulsion or severely shattered kidney, reconstruction may

be impossible, and nephrectomy may be required to save the patient's life [5].

Relative indications for renal exploration include incomplete staging, devitalized renal parenchyma, vascular injury, and urinary extravasation [6]. In a hemodynamically unstable patient, radiographic assessment is not possible before laparotomy and an unexpected retroperitoneal hematoma may be found at the time of laparotomy in the trauma patient. At this time, if the patient's clinical condition permits, a single abdominal radiograph (imaging the kidneys, ureter and bladder) taken 10 minutes after the bolus administration of 2 cc/kg of intravenous contrast, delivered as a bolus ("one-shot" intravenous pyelogram (IVP)), in a normotensive patient, is helpful [7]. This film is most helpful for confirming the presence of a normally functioning contralateral kidney and may occasionally help to diagnose the injury in the affected renal unit. All patients with penetrating trauma and incomplete preoperative staging and a retroperitoneal hematoma require exploration. Although the one-shot IVP

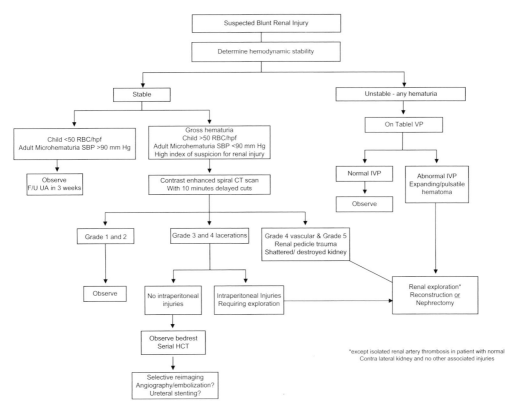

Fig. 2. Management algorithms for blunt renal injury. *Abbreviations:* RBC, red blood cells; hpf, high power field. (*Adapted from* Santucci RA, Wessells H, Bartsch G, et al. Evaluation and management of renal injuries: consensus statement of the Renal Trauma Subcommittee. BJU Int 2004;93:937.).

may be indeterminate, a recent study found that it successfully obviated renal exploration in 32% of patients in whom it was required [7]. Furthermore, this approach has not been found to increase the rate of unnecessary nephrectomy [3]. The initial laparotomy is the best time for any required renal reconstruction. Delayed exploration has resulted in nephrectomy rates as high as 50% [4].

Operative technique

The main steps related to exploring an injured kidney and, if necessary, reconstructing a kidney include staging the injury, controlling renal hemorrhage, preserving maximal renal parenchyma, and reducing potential complications attributable to the injured kidney. Historically, renal exploration in the trauma setting usually resulted in total nephrectomy. Today, however, through a refined approach to proximal vascular control and a meticulous approach to reconstruction, most injured

kidneys requiring surgical exploration can be salvaged [3,8–15].

Importance of proximal vascular control

Unplanned nephrectomy in the trauma setting stems from uncontrolled hemorrhage. While the literature shows disagreement about the need for proximal control [15–19], the prudent course is to routinely obtain proximal vascular control before opening the retroperitoneal hematoma. While temporary vascular occlusion is rarely necessary (approximately 17% of renal explorations at San Francisco General Hospital), no accurate method has been found to determine which kidneys will require this maneuver during subsequent reconstruction. Some researchers have suggested that pedicle control can be safely obtained following release of the perinephric hematoma. However, their reports about such cases have shown nephrectomy rates approximately three times higher than those with early vascular control [15,20,21].

Table 1
The American Association for the Surgery of Trauma
(AAST) organ injury severity scale for renal trauma

Grade	Injury	Description
I	Contusion	Microscopic or gross hematuria; urological studies normal
	Hematoma	Subcapsular, nonexpanding without parenchymal laceration
II	Haematoma	Nonexpanding perirenal hematoma confined to renal retroperitoneum
	Laceration	<1 cm parenchymal depth of renal cortex without urinary extravasation
III	Laceration	>1 cm depth of renal cortex, without collecting system rupture or urinary extravasation
IV	Laceration	Parenchymal laceration extending through the renal cortex, medulla, and collecting system (meaning extravasation)
	Vascular	Main renal artery or vein injury with contained hemorrhage
V	Laceration	Completely shattered kidney
	Vascular	Avulsion of renal hilum which devascularizes kidney

The injury scale is advanced one grade for bilateral
injuries up to Grade III.

The traumatized kidney should be explored
through a midline transperitoneal incision extending from the xiphoid process to the pubic symphysis. The cephalad extent of the incision must
be as large as possible so that the renal injury can
be easily seen. Except in cases of renal pedicle
avulsion, all associated intra-abdominal injuries
(ie, injuries to spleen, liver, pancreas, small and
large intestine) should be addressed before renal
exploration. This method allows Gerota's fascia
to maintain its natural tamponade effect on the
hematoma.

Operative technique

The approach to the injured kidney begins with
proximal vascular control. If enough personnel
are available, handheld retractors, such as

Richardson or Deaver retractors, can be deployed
rapidly and are sufficient to impart visualization.
If not, then a self-retaining retractor, such as
a Bookwalter retractor, should be used. Following
visualization, the transverse colon should be
wrapped in moist laparotomy sponges and placed
on the chest. Then the small intestine should be
placed in a bowel bag or moist sponges and
retracted superiorly onto the right chest (Fig. 4).
This exposes the root of the mesentery and the ligament of Treitz and the underlying great vessels.
The retroperitoneal incision should be made
over the aorta superior to the inferior mesenteric
artery, and extending up to the ligament of Treitz
(Fig. 5). If a large retroperitoneal hematoma obvi-
ates easy palpation of the aorta at the level of the
ligament of Treitz, the incision may be made medial to the visualized inferior mesenteric vein. This
vein is an important guide, running a few centi-
meters left of the aorta. The vein is easily identifi-
able, even in the presence of a large hematoma.
Dissection should be carried superiorly along the
anterior wall of the aorta until the left renal vein
is identified crossing anterior to the aorta. The
left renal vein is encircled but not occluded with
a vessel loop, allowing for retraction. Now, the
left renal vein serves as a guide to the remaining
renal vessels, each of which is then secured with
vessel loops in the following order: Left renal
vein, left renal artery, right renal vein, right renal
artery. The average time for this proximal renal vascular control, even at a training institution, is 12 minutes. These vessels are all left unoccluded unless
heavy bleeding is encountered during the renal dissection. In the authors' experience, most bleeding is
successfully controlled with manual compression
alone. Temporary renal vascular occlusion should
be kept below 30 minutes to minimize warm ischemic damage. After vascular control has been successfully achieved, the injured kidney may be
exposed by mobilizing the ipsilateral colon along
the white line of Toldt and reflecting it medially.
Gerota's fascia is then incised along the lateral aspect of the kidney to completely expose the kidney.
Care should be taken to maintain the integrity of
the renal capsule as the kidney is mobilized to
decrease hemorrhage and preserve the capsule for
later closure.

Parenchymal injuries

Significant amounts of devitalized renal parenchyma are often best managed by early surgical
debridement. Expectant management of patients

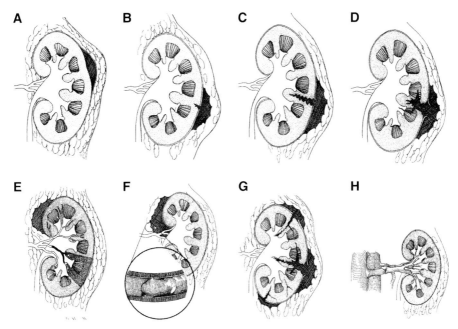

Fig. 3. Renal injuries as classified by the American Association for the Society of Trauma (AAST) organ injury scale. (A) A Grade 1 injury is a contusion or a contained subcapsular hematoma without parenchymal laceration. (B) A Grade 2 injury is a nonexpanding, confined perirenal hematoma or cortical laceration <1 cm deep, without urinary extravasation. (C) A Grade 3 injury is a parenchymal laceration extending >1 cm into the cortex, but without urinary extravasation. (D) A Grade 4 injury can be a parenchymal or a vascular injury. Parenchymal Grade 4 injuries are those with a laceration extending through the corticomedullary junction and into the collecting system. A segmental vessel may also be lacerated. (E) A Grade 4 vascular injury consists of a segmental renal artery thrombosis without a parenchymal laceration. Renal arteries are end-arteries and the area of parenchyma subtended by the injured segmental artery will be ischemic. (F) Grade 5 injuries are multiple and consist of shattered kidneys, pedicle avulsion, or main renal artery thrombosis. These injuries are by nature life-threatening. Main renal artery thrombosis is generally due to intimal disruption with resultant thrombosis, as shown in the close-up of the figure. (G) A Grade 5 injury can also be a "shattered" kidney, consisting of multiple major lacerations. (H) Avulsion of the main renal artery or main renal vein is also a Grade 5 injury. (*Adapted from* Nash PA, Carroll PR. Staging of renal trauma. In: McAninch JW, editor. Traumatic and reconstructive urology. Philadelphia: W.B. Saunders; 1996.)

with devitalized fragments and associated intra-abdominal injury may lead to a higher rate of abscess and infected urinoma formation as well as delayed complications [22]. Data indicate that immediate exploration in this setting reduces the post-trauma complication rate from 82% to 23%. [23]. This result suggests that major renal lacerations with devitalized fragments and associated intra-abdominal injuries should be immediately repaired, particularly if a laparotomy is already planned by the trauma surgeon. Additionally, patients with a major devitalized fragment associated with urinary extravasation and a significant hematoma are ultimately best treated by early exploration and reconstruction, even without concomitant intraperitoneal injury. However, the nonoperative approach in this situation may be more prudent for the urologist who rarely

undertakes renal exploration in the trauma setting, as the chance of unnecessary nephrectomy is increased.

Urinary extravasation signifies collecting system violation secondary to a major renal laceration, but does not specifically mandate surgical repair. The collecting system may be disrupted at a fornix, a minor or major calyx, or even through the renal pelvis and ureteropelvic junction (UPJ). While the majority of lacerations into fornices and minor calyces will seal spontaneously, larger degrees of extravasation may leak for a prolonged period and are less likely to resolve spontaneously [24]. Serial CT scans are critical in the management of patients with large degrees of extravasation. The first scan should be obtained at approximately 36 to 48 hours post-injury to rule out the development of significant new

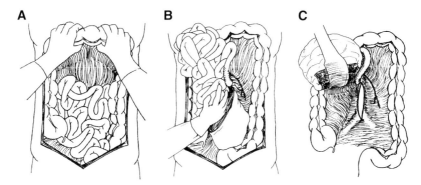

Fig. 4. Optimal exposure for proximal vascular control. (*A*) A midline laparotomy, extending from xiphoid to pubis should be made, if not already made by the trauma surgeons. Ensure that the superior extent of the incision is as high up as possible. The first maneuver is to place the transverse colon onto the chest. (*B*) The small bowel is reflected out of the body toward the right nipple. (*C*) Small bowel contents are placed into a bowel bag or covered in moist laparotomy pads. The root of the small bowel mesentery should be visible, allowing for excellent visualization of the posterior peritoneal incision overlying the aorta from the ligament of Treitz to the aortic bifurcation. (*From* Brandes SB, McAninch JW. Surgical exposure and repair of the traumatized kidney. Atlas of Urol Clin North Am 1998;6(2):32–33.)

complications. Intervention is indicated in the setting of sepsis, ongoing leakage, or significant urinoma formation. In these cases, placement of an indwelling ureteral stent or even a nephrostomy tube may speed resolution of extravasation. Lacerations of the renal pelvis usually do not resolve spontaneously and should be surgically repaired. Similarly, UPJ avulsion mandates surgical repair. These unusual injuries are more commonly found in the setting of deceleration injury or in children, but may also take place in adults with an undiagnosed congenital anomaly, such as ureteropelvic junction obstruction. CT findings that suggest UPJ avulsion include nonvisualization of the ipsilateral ureter and medial extravasation of contrast material [25]. The urologist should also maintain a low threshold for repair of an extravasating kidney associated with a gunshot wound. These wounds are often associated with significant devitalized parenchyma secondary to blast effect, especially when a high-velocity missile has been used.

Principles of reconstruction

For all renal reconstructions, eight general steps apply:

1. The entire kidney must be broadly exposed.
2. Measures for temporary vascular occlusion must be taken to stop bleeding not arrested by manual compression of the parenchyma.
3. Nonviable parenchyma must be sharply debrided.

4. Hemostasis must be established and meticulously maintained.
5. The collecting system closure must be made watertight.
6. After renorrhaphy, the parenchymal defect must be covered by reapproximation of the parenchymal edges.
7. The omental interposition flap must be placed to separate the reconstructed kidney from surrounding pancreatic, colonic, or vascular injuries.
8. The retroperitoneal drain must be put in place.

The kidney should be debrided sharply back to viable, bleeding parenchyma. Approximately 30% of one normally functioning kidney is required to avoid dialysis. This rule of thumb may serve as a guide in determining whether renal salvage should be undertaken. Major polar injuries are best managed with partial nephrectomy (Fig. 6), while lacerations to the mid-kidney should undergo renorrhaphy (Fig. 7). For hemostasis, the arterial vessels should be individually suture-ligated with 4-0 chromic sutures. To assist hemostasis, place hemostatic agents, such as thrombin-soaked absorbable gelatin sponge bolsters, between the cut parenchymal edges. Then inspect the collecting system for obvious tears. To better find any openings, inject 2 to 3 cc methylene blue into the renal pelvis using a 27-gauge needle. Tears are then oversewn with running 4-0 chromic suture. A stent is placed only in cases of significant renal pelvis or ureteral injuries, but not in simple

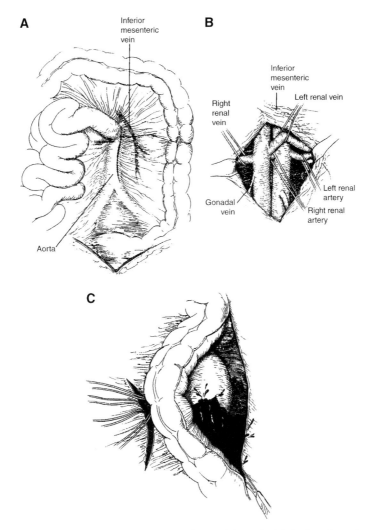

Fig. 5. Surgical approach to the renal vessels and kidney. The overlying principle is that of proximal vascular control. (*A*) The posterior peritoneum is incised over the aorta medial to the inferior mesenteric vein. (*B*) The renal vessels are isolated with vessel loops to secure, but not occlude, the vessels. This should be done in the following order: Left renal vein, left renal artery, right renal vein, right renal artery. (*C*) After the renal vessels are secured, an incision is made in the posterior peritoneum lateral to the colon, exposing the kidney. (*From* McAninch JW. Surgery for renal trauma. In: Novick AC, Pontes ES, Streem SB, editors. Stewart's operative urology, 2nd edition. Baltimore (MD): Williams and Wilkins; 1989. p. 235–6.)

calyceal injuries. For a deep, slit-like parenchymal laceration from a knife or sword, the thin parenchymal defect will not permit easy access to the collecting system, and urologists rely on closure of the overlying parenchyma to seal the collecting system.

If the renal capsule is intact and viable, it should be used without tension as the primary means to close the parenchymal defect. If the capsule has been destroyed or the defect is too large to close primarily without causing ischemia, an omental flap can be used. The omentum, once guided through the paracolic gutter to reach the kidney, can be sutured to the defect. If the omentum is not available, the defect may be covered with perinephric fat or a peritoneal free graft. However, these are less desirable options. In the case of a shattered kidney or multiple deep lacerations, the kidney may be placed in an envelope of Vicryl mesh to stabilize the repair.

A LOWER POLE LACERATION

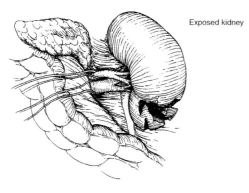

Exposed kidney

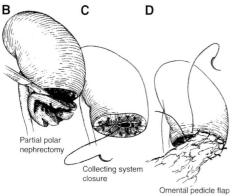

B   **C**   **D**

Partial polar
nephrectomy

Collecting system
closure

Omental pedicle flap

Fig. 6. Partial nephrectomy technique following lower pole laceration. (*A*) Exposed kidney. The kidney is totally mobilized to completely assess for injury. The ureter is carefully inspected. (*B*) Partial polar nephrectomy. The nonviable renal tissue is meticulously removed. Hemostasis is obtained with manual compression of the kidney during this maneuver. (*C*) Collecting system closure. The collecting system is closed with absorbable suture and discrete end-arteries are oversewn. (*D*) Omental pedical flap. Defect coverage is done with omentum, or alternatively, with residual capsule if it was preserved. (*From* McAninch JW. Surgery for renal trauma. In: Novick AC, Pontes ES, Streem SB, editors. Stewart's operative urology, 2nd edition. Baltimore (MD): Williams and Wilkins; 1989. p. 237.)

Following reconstruction involving the collecting system, a Penrose drain is placed adjacent to the kidney and connected to a urostomy bag to drain any leak if necessary. Alternatively, a suction drain may be used, as long as it is not connected to suction because suction prolongs urinary drainage. These drains are typically removed after 48 to 72 hours unless output is high, in which case the drainage creatinine should be measured. If the creatinine value suggests a urine leak, the drain should be left in place for a longer period. Placement of an indwelling ureteral stent may help to expedite sealing of a persistent urine leak.

Vascular injuries

Renovascular injuries are uncommon. In a survey of patients over a 16-year period at six major trauma centers, only 89 patients were found to have renovascular injury [26]. Most injuries are to the renal artery only (60%), followed by the renal vein (30%), followed by a combination of arterial and venous injury (10%) [27]. Physical examination is not usually specific. Major injury to the main renal artery or vein almost invariably requires operative management. Unlike parenchymal lacerations, renovascular injuries are frequently impossible to repair, and may result in nephrectomy. Proximal vascular control is particularly critical in these cases and, indeed, temporary vascular occlusion can be accomplished without any resultant negative sequelae in 90% of patients [8]. These patients have higher rates of complications, renal loss, and mortality when compared with those with nonvascular renal injuries [9].

Arterial injury

CT findings consistent with main renal artery injury include lack of renal enhancement or abrupt cut-off of an enhancing artery. Segmental arterial injuries typically appear as wedge-shaped infarcts with the apex facing the renal hilum. Injuries to the main renal vein typically appear as central or large hematomas, which may displace the kidney anteriorly. Vascular injuries typically occur secondary to deceleration trauma causing the disruption of the inelastic intimal layer with subsequent irreversible parenchymal ischemia and infarction.

Despite the ongoing advances in trauma care, successful renal salvage after major renovascular injury only occurs in 25% to 35% of cases, at best [26]. Time to reperfusion is the major factor in determining the outcome. Renal function is significantly impaired following 3 hours of total and 6 hours of partial ischemia [28]. Despite technically successful repair, late hypertension occurs in approximately 50% of renal arterial injuries managed nonoperatively, compared with 57% that were revascularized. Renal arterial repair should thus be reserved for solitary kidneys, bilaterally injured kidneys, and in the rare situation of

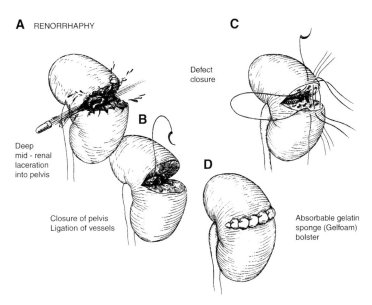

Fig. 7. Renorrhaphy technique. (*A*) Deep mid-renal laceration into pelvis, with collecting system entry. (*B*) Closure of pelvis, ligation of vessels. Sharp debridement is performed to viable tissue edges. Following this, the collecting system is closed with absorbable suture and discrete end-arteries are suture-ligated. (*C*) Defect closure. Interrupted polyglactin 2-0 sutures are placed into the renal capsule. After these are placed, thrombin-soaked absorbable gelatin sponges are placed as bolsters into the defect. (*D*) Absorbable gelatin sponge bolster. The parenchyma is approximated by tying the capsular sutures loosely so that they do not rip through the capsule. (*From* McAninch JW. Surgery for renal trauma. In: Novick AC, Pontes ES, Streem SB, editors. Stewart's operative urology, 2nd edition. Baltimore (MD): Williams and Wilkins; 1989. p. 238.)

detection within 6 hours of injury. Endovascular stenting may have a limited role, as maintaining patency requires anticoagulation, which is rarely possible in the traumatically injured patient, especially with polytrauma to the spleen or liver. If detection of renal artery thrombosis is delayed and laparotomy is otherwise indicated, nephrectomy should be performed. Otherwise, the kidney may be allowed to atrophy, with delayed nephrectomy performed if hypertension develops.

In cases of main renal artery injury, the type of repair indicated relates to the extent and mechanism of injury. Penetrating injuries with incomplete transection may be primarily repaired using 5-0 prolene sutures. Blunt injuries typically require thrombectomy and debridement of the damaged arterial segment. Ideally, a primary tension-free reanastomosis of the injured artery should be undertaken. If this is not feasible, the authors recommend an interposition vascular graft. Ex-vivo renal reconstruction and autotransplantation into the iliac fossa are rarely indicated in the critically injured patient with multiple associated injuries. However, such procedures are technically feasible and have been reported

[29]. Segmental arterial injuries may be safely ligated, with few complications arising from the subsequently devascularized renal parenchyma. Alternatively, a partially lacerated segmental artery may be repaired with 5-0 or 6-0 prolene suture.

Venous injury

Injury to the main renal vein typically results in significant hemorrhage and may require ligation. If reconstruction is feasible, the partially lacerated vein may be repaired with 5-0 prolene suture following appropriate vascular clamping (Fig. 8). Injuries to segmental veins may be safely ligated because of the extensive renal venous collateral circulation.

Postoperative care

A urethral catheter should be maintained until the patient is hemodynamically stable and mobile enough to void. The patient should be kept on bed rest until gross hematuria clears. The authors recommend obtaining an abdominal CT scan and a radionuclide renal scan (DMSA scan) at

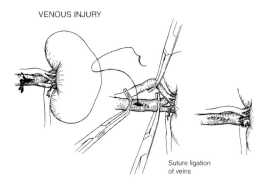

Fig. 8. Renovascular injury repair. Venous injuries can occur in the segmental renal veins or the main renal vein itself. Primary venorrhaphy of a main renal vein injury. Ligation of segmental renal vein injuries may be done without compromise of kidney function. (*From* McAninch JW. Surgery for renal trauma. In: Novick AC, Pontes ES, Streem SB, editors. Stewart's operative urology, 2nd edition. Baltimore (MD): Williams and Wilkins; 1989. p. 239.)

approximately 3 months to quantify the function of the injured or reconstructed kidney. In measuring the function of traumatically injured and subsequently reconstructed kidneys, the authors found that the average differential renal function of the repaired kidney was 39%, which corresponds to about two thirds of the full renal function of a single healthy kidney.

References

[1] Santucci RA, McAninch JW, Safir M, et al. Validation of the American Association for the Surgery of Trauma organ injury severity scale for the kidney. J Trauma 2001;50:195.

[2] Santucci RA, McAninch JM. Grade IV renal injuries: evaluation, treatment, and outcome. World J Surg 2001;25:1565.

[3] McAninch JW, Carroll PR, Klosterman PW, et al. Renal reconstruction after injury. J Urol 1991;145:932.

[4] Holcroft JW, Trunkey DD, Minagi H, et al. Renal trauma and retroperitoneal hematomas-indications for exploration. J Trauma 1975;15:1045.

[5] Nash PA, Bruce JE, McAninch JW. Nephrectomy for traumatic renal injuries. J Urol 1995;153:609.

[6] Meng MV, Brandes SB, McAninch JW. Renal trauma: indications and techniques for surgical exploration. World J Urol 1999;17:71.

[7] Morey AF, McAninch JW, Tiller BK, et al. Single shot intraoperative excretory urography for the immediate evaluation of renal trauma. J Urol 1999; 161:1088.

[8] Carroll PR, McAninch JW, Wong A, et al. Outcome after temporary vascular occlusion for the management of renal trauma. J Urol 1994;151:1171.

[9] Carroll PR, McAninch JW, Klosterman P, et al. Renovascular trauma: risk assessment, surgical management, and outcome. J Trauma 1990;30:547.

[10] McAninch JW, Carroll PR. Renal exploration after trauma. Indications and reconstructive techniques. Urol Clin North Am 1989;16:203.

[11] Carroll PR, Klosterman P, McAninch JW. Early vascular control for renal trauma: a critical review. J Urol 1989;141:826.

[12] Carroll PR, McAninch JW. Staging of renal trauma. Urol Clin North Am 1989;16:193.

[13] Carroll PR, Klosterman PW, McAninch JW. Surgical management of renal trauma: analysis of risk factors, technique, and outcome. J Trauma 1988; 28:1071.

[14] Carroll PR, McAninch JW. Operative indications in penetrating renal trauma. J Trauma 1985;25:587.

[15] McAninch JW, Carroll PR. Renal trauma: kidney preservation through improved vascular control—a refined approach. J Trauma 1982;22:285.

[16] Santucci RA, Wessells H, Bartsch G, et al. Evaluation and management of renal injuries: consensus statement of the renal trauma subcommittee. BJU Int 2004;93:937.

[17] Sahin H, Akay AF, Yilmaz G, et al. Retrospective analysis of 135 renal trauma cases. Int J Urol 2004; 11:332.

[18] Heyns CF. Renal trauma: indications for imaging and surgical exploration. BJU Int 2004;93:1165.

[19] Nicol AJ, Theunissen D. Renal salvage in penetrating kidney injuries: a prospective analysis. J Trauma 2002;53:351.

[20] Nash PA, McAninch JW, Bruce JE, et al. Sonourethrography in the evaluation of anterior urethral strictures. J Urol 1995;154:72.

[21] Corriere JN Jr, McAndrew JD, Benson GS. Intraoperative decision-making in renal trauma surgery. J Trauma 1991;31:1390.

[22] Husmann DA, Morris JS. Attempted nonoperative management of blunt renal lacerations extending through the corticomedullary junction: the short-term and long-term sequelae. J Urol 1990; 143:682.

[23] Husmann DA, Gilling PJ, Perry MO, et al. Major renal lacerations with a devitalized fragment following blunt abdominal trauma: a comparison between nonoperative (expectant) versus surgical management. J Urol 1774;1993:150.

[24] Matthews LA, Smith EM, Spirnak JP. Nonoperative treatment of major blunt renal lacerations with urinary extravasation. J Urol 1997;157:2056.

[25] Townsend M, DeFalco AJ. Absence of ureteral opacification below ureteral disruption: a sentinel CT finding. AJR Am J Roentgenol 1995;164:253.

[26] Knudson MM, Harrison PB, Hoyt DB, et al. Outcome after major renovascular injuries: a Western Trauma Association multicenter report. J Trauma 2000;49:1116.

[27] Clark DE, Georgitis JW, Ray FS. Renal arterial injuries caused by blunt trauma. Surgery 1981;90:87.

[28] McAninch JW. Traumatic and reconstructive urology. Philadelphia: W.B. Saunders; 1996.

[29] Fay R, Brosman S, Lindstrom R, et al. Renal artery thrombosis: a successful revascularization by auto-transplantation. J Urol 1974;111:572.

ELSEVIER
SAUNDERS

Urol Clin N Am 33 (2006) 33–40

UROLOGIC
CLINICS
of North America

The Diagnosis, Management, and Outcomes of Pediatric Renal Injuries

Jill C. Buckley, MD[a,b], Jack W. McAninch, MD[a,b],*

[a]Department of Urology, University of California School of Medicine, San Francisco, CA, USA
[b]Urology Service, San Francisco General Hospital, 1001 Potrero Avenue, San Francisco, CA 94110, USA

Over the past 20 years the management of pediatric trauma has largely shifted to conservative management including most pediatric renal trauma [1,2]. The kidney is frequently injured in pediatric blunt abdominal trauma [3,4], with an injury occurring 10% to 20% of the time [3,5,6]. The lack of perirenal fat, relatively larger size of the pediatric kidney in relation to the rest of the body, and decreased protection from the more pliable, less ossified pediatric thoracic cage are possible explanations for why children are more susceptible to renal injuries [7,8].

Blunt trauma accounts for approximately 90% of pediatric renal injuries with the remainder caused by a penetrating injury [8,9]. Most pediatric renal trauma is minor requiring no intervention with minimal risk of a future complication. It is the small proportion of children who sustain a severe potentially life-threatening renal injury who need immediate assessment and management [9,10]. The challenge lies in early detection and selective management of severe grade IV to V renal injuries because obvious clinical signs are not always present. Taking into consideration the hemodynamic stability of the child, mechanism of injury, associated nonrenal injuries, radiographic CT or intravenous pyelogram staging, and clinical examination, appropriate operative versus nonoperative management can be selected with an expected (>98%) high renal salvage rate [2,9].

Initial diagnosis

As in all trauma patients, the first goal is to quickly assess the situation and stabilize the pediatric patient. If the child is hemodynamically unstable or has suffered a severe intra-abdominal penetrating injury, immediate operative exploration is the standard of care. Not every penetrating renal trauma mandates operative exploration (ie, an isolated renal stab wound) but the onus lies on the treating physician to prove the child can be safely managed nonoperatively through appropriate renal staging [9,11,12]. In hemodynamically stable children, who do not meet trauma criteria for immediate operative exploration, a thorough medical history and evaluation should ensue. Especially important is a detailed report of the mechanism of injury because this in itself may prompt further evaluation and provide insight into the transfer of energy responsible for the renal injury [13,14].

A systematic approach can be used in every pediatric (and adult) trauma evaluation. At the initial evaluation five main areas should be addressed (Box 1). To help guide the initial work-up and determine the appropriate management to achieve optimal renal preservation a pediatric renal trauma algorithm is provided (Fig. 1) [9].

Hemodynamic stability

The hemodynamic state of a child is a difficult parameter to interpret at the initial evaluation because of a child's ability to maintain blood pressure despite severe hypovolemia [15,16]. On the rare occasion severe hypotension is present, immediate surgical exploration is warranted. Unlike in adult patients, where shock is a sensitive

* Corresponding author.
  E-mail address: jmcaninch@urol.ucsf.edu
(J.W. McAninch).

> **Box 1. Initial evaluation: five core criteria**
>
> 1. Hemodynamic stability
> 2. Type or mechanism of trauma
> 3. Associated nonrenal injuries
> 4. Hematuria
> 5. Clinical examination

indicator of hypovolemia (systolic blood pressure <90 mm Hg), such is not the case in children; it is important to perform serial clinical examinations, hematocrits, and blood pressures in all children who sustain significant trauma. Some level I trauma centers have adopted an ICU protocol for any child undergoing nonoperative management of a severe renal injury. It mandates the child be placed on bed rest for a minimum of 24 to 48 hours to allow continual monitoring of their hemodynamic state, hematocrit, and clinical examination [2,9]. If any significant change should occur (ie, a drop in hematocrit unresponsive to 3 U of packed red blood cells or enlarging flank ecchymosis), repeat CT imaging or renal exploration should occur depending on the clinical situation to reassess the injury. It is usually in the first 24 to 48 hours that hemodynamic instability occurs, although delayed bleeding should always be a consideration in a child with a severe renal injury.

Mechanism of injury and associated injuries

There are three main reasons pediatric renal trauma patients undergo immediate exploration: (1) hemodynamic instability, (2) a penetrating injury, or (3) associated nonrenal injuries requiring operative exploration. Trauma surgeons at many institutions explore penetrating abdominal injuries because of an inability to detect visceral injuries adequately. Renal exploration is performed concurrently to stage the renal injury and reconstruct the kidney in stable patients as the benefits of nonoperative management are lost [9,17,18].

In the event of an isolated penetrating renal injury in a hemodynamically stable child, selective nonoperative management can be used but only after complete CT staging [9,12]. The role of nonoperative management continues to expand as experience and comfort grow with observational management of penetrating trauma.

Penetrating injuries represent a minority of the pediatric renal trauma. Approximately 90% are the result of blunt trauma [9,19]. Accidents (ie, motor vehicle, pedestrian, and falls) account for most pediatric renal trauma (Table 1). In

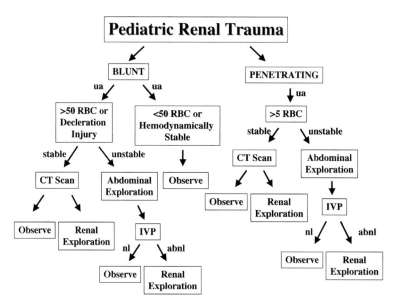

Fig. 1. Algorithm for pediatric renal trauma management. abnl, abnormal; IVP, intravenous pyelogram; nl, normal; RBC, red blood cell; ua, urine analysis. (*From* Buckley JC, McAninch JW. Pediatric renal injuries: management guidelines from a 25-year experience. J Urol 2004;172:687; with permission.)

Table 1
Mechanism of injury in 333 pediatric blunt renal trauma patients

Mechanism	percentage of total
Pedestrian accident	33
Motor vehicle accident	32
Fall	14
Motorcycle accident	13
Assault	7
Other	1

Data from Buckley JC, McAninch JW. Pediatric renal injuries: Management guidelines from a 25-year experience. J Unl 2004;172:687; with permission.

hemodynamically stable children, the mechanism of injury (blunt versus penetrating) becomes important in the initial assessment and criteria for radiographic imaging (see hematuria section below). Unlike penetrating trauma, most blunt pediatric renal trauma is successfully managed nonoperatively because of accurate CT grading and staging [2,9,16,20,21]. Undisputed in the literature is the conservative management of grade I to III renal injuries (Fig. 2) [22]. Many series in the literature also support selective nonoperative management of blunt grade IV renal injuries with some extending nonoperative management to include grade V renal injuries [2,5,6,9,23].

Unique to blunt renal trauma is a deceleration injury that causes a shearing force on the fixed renal hilum [8,13,14]. All children who sustain a deceleration injury (ie, fall or motor vehicle accident) should undergo CT imaging to assess the renal hilum even in the absence of microhematuria or gross hematuria [16,24]. The force of impact on the renal hilum may result in a main renal artery thrombosis, main renal vessel avulsion, or ureteral pelvic junction dismemberment [25].

Hematuria

Dip stick analysis or formal urine analysis should be performed at the initial evaluation as a screening tool for additional imaging [9,22,26]. Two important points need to be emphasized with regards to hematuria. First, hematuria screening is performed to guide the need for additional imaging based on the number of red blood cells per high powered field and type of blunt versus penetrating trauma (> 50 red blood cells per high powered field in blunt trauma and > 5 red blood cells per high powered field in penetrating trauma [Table 2]) [9,24,27]. Second, the degree of renal injury cannot be determined by the presence or absence, or the amount, of hematuria. Several series have reported gross hematuria in minor renal injuries and minimal or no hematuria

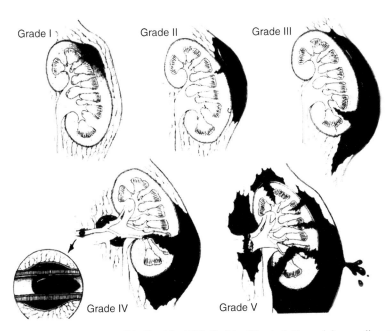

Fig. 2. Renal injury grades. (*From* Moore EE, Shackford SR, Pachter HL, et al. Organ injury scaling: spleen, liver, and kidney. J Trauma 1989;29:1664; with permission.)

Table 2
Hematuria vis-a-vis grade in 374 pediatric renal injuries

Urinalysis results (rbc/hpf)[a]	Grade				
	I	II	III	IV	V
Blunt injuries (N = 333)					
Not done	4	—	—	—	—
Absent	1	—	1	—	—
0–2	16	—	—	1	—
2–5	43	—	—	—	—
5–10	51	—	—	—	—
10–20	38	—	—	—	—
20–50	33	1	—	1	—
50–100	24	—	—	—	—
Too numerous to count	45	—	—	1	—
Gross hematuria	53	8	3	8	1
Total	308	9	4	11	1
Penetrating injuries (N = 41)					
Not done	—	1	—	—	—
Absent	1	—	—	—	—
0–2	—	1	—	—	—
2–5	—	—	—	1	—
5–10	2	—	2	—	—
10–20	1	—	2	—	—
20–50	1	—	—	1	—
50–100	2	1	1	—	—
Too numerous to count	1	—	—	—	—
Gross hematuria	4	1	9	9	—
Total	12	4	14	11	0

Data from Buckley JC, McAninch JW. Pediatric renal injuries: Management guidelines from a 25-year experience. J Urol 2004;172:687; with permission.

[a] Red blood cells per high-power field.

in severe renal grade IV and V renal injuries (see Table 2) [9,24,28]. An isolated finding of microhematuria of <50 red blood cells per high powered field in a blunt pediatric renal trauma does not alone meet the criteria for CT imaging (see Fig. 1) [9,24,27].

Clinical examination

Every pediatric renal trauma should undergo a complete trauma evaluation. An unstable child requires immediate resuscitation and possible operative exploration. If the child is stable, a thorough secondary examination should be done to ensure no injuries are missed. Signs or symptoms that may suggest a renal injury in a child are complaints of flank, abdominal, or pelvic pain; a tender or fractured rib; flank or abdominal ecchymosis (ie, seat belt sign); or gross hematuria. Any of these findings should prompt CT imaging [9,11].

Staging

Nonoperative management of renal trauma including pediatric renal trauma has been made possible by the accurate staging and grading of renal injuries by CT imaging. The detailed anatomic imaging of the retroperitoneal and peritoneal cavities allows the surgeon to make an informed management decision based on the grade of renal injury and the associated nonurologic injuries. A renal protocol CT scan consisting of noncontrast, contrast, and delayed phases allows for evaluation of the renal vasculature, parenchyma, and collecting system, respectively [29,30]. CT imaging is the standard of care based on its accuracy and ability to diagnose both urologic and nonurologic abdominal and pelvic injuries [3,31]. When preoperative renal CT staging cannot be performed (ie, the patient is undergoing immediate exploration), a single-shot intravenous pyelogram (2 mL/kg of intravenous bolus) [30] should be performed to identify and document a normal contralateral kidney in the event a nephrectomy is performed. Additionally, it may provide information on the function of the kidney in question and limit the amount of exploration necessary.

If neither a CT scan nor an intraoperative one-shot intravenous pyelogram is available, the renal injury can be staged at the operative exploration. If a large, expanding, or pulsatile hematoma is identified in the retroperitoneum, vascular control should be obtained before renal exploration (as described by McAninch and coworkers [14,32]) to avoid needless nephrectomies secondary to uncontrollable bleeding.

Selective management

With the widespread use of CT imaging to stage and grade renal injuries, selective management of each child can occur to achieve optimal renal salvage with minimal morbidity. The American Association for the Surgery of Trauma (AAST) organ injury severity scale is the most widely used and validated grading system for renal trauma (see Fig. 2) [22,31]. All hemodynamically stable grade I to III injuries can be managed nonoperatively with spontaneous healing of the renal injury demonstrated on follow-up CT imaging or renal functional scans [2,9,20,23]. A grade I renal injury (renal contusion) without gross hematuria can be discharged home without further imaging and followed-up with urinalysis. Any patient with gross hematuria or grade II to III renal injuries should be admitted to the hospital for a minimum of 24 hours and placed on bed rest and observation because the risk of bleeding is the highest during this time period. Low-grade fevers can be seen with hematomas and need not prompt further evaluation or intervention. Once the gross hematuria has resolved, the child can be discharged home with strict instructions to avoid all strenuous activity until repeat imaging has documented complete healing [9,20]. No further imaging is necessary as along as appropriate healing and function is demonstrated; however, the child should be monitored clinically for late posttraumatic renal complications, such as hypertension.

Severe renal injuries (grade IV–V) require careful selective management based on hemodynamic stability, mechanism of injury, associated nonrenal injuries, and clinical presentation to determine operative versus nonoperative management. Children who are hemodynamically unstable or sustain a severe penetrating intra-abdominal injury should undergo immediate operative exploration (see Fig. 1). At the time of operative exploration, a one-shot intravenous pyelogram (2 mL/kg intravenous bolus) [30] should be performed to document a functional contralateral kidney and provide additional information on the condition of the injured kidney [9,30]. The high association (30%–80%) of significant nonurologic injuries in severe grade IV to V renal injuries often drives operative exploration, precluding nonoperative management [2,5,9,20,27].

The remaining hemodynamically stable children who have been staged by CT imaging and followed with consecutive stable hematocrits can be admitted to the ICU for strict bed rest and clinical monitoring with an excellent prognosis. Aggressive nonoperative management requires close observation, serial examinations and hematocrits, and strict bed rest. Repeat CT imaging should be performed routinely at 48 hours or earlier if prompted by a clinical change to reassess the injury. As long as the child remains hemodynamically stable (with or without blood transfusions), and the CT scan demonstrates a stable hematoma or amount of urinary extravasation, observation may continue [2,9,11]. If the child at any point demonstrates hemodynamic instability (hypovolemia or is unresponsive to 3 U of packed red blood cells), they should be surgically explored for persistent bleeding or be considered for

angiography and embolization of bleeding renal vessels [11].

Angioembolization of selective segmental renal arteries has been successful and is particularly useful for primary treatment of isolated grade IV renal injuries with segmental artery bleeding or delayed bleeding in grades II to IV injuries [33,34]. As in delayed bleeding after a partial nephrectomy, the patient should be stabilized with blood transfusions and then taken to interventional radiology for angioembolization. Although this is an attractive alternative to surgical exploration, this should only be done by an experienced interventional radiologist in a non–renal failure patient with a definable segmental artery injury.

Symptomatic or worsening urinary extravasation demonstrated on repeat CT imaging can be managed either with percutaneous drainage or internal ureteral stenting with confirmed resolution of extravasation on follow-up imaging (Fig. 3) [6,35,36]. Experience is growing with pediatric endoscopic placement of ureteral stents and it has emerged as a successful way to manage large urinomas resulting from grade IV laceration injuries [37]. If minimally invasive management is chosen by percutaneous or internal drainage (ureteral double J stent) urethral catheter drainage is recommended. With delayed intervention rates reported between 25% and 50% in the literature for severe pediatric renal injuries, conservative management should be reserved to institutions that can provide appropriate resources (ie, a skilled interventional radiology team or access to pediatric endoscopic equipment) [5,6,20,37,38]. For conservative management to be successful in severe renal injuries the treating surgeon needs to be proactive in monitoring and adjusting treatment.

If improving, the child can be transferred to the pediatric ward after 48 hours of ICU monitoring and repeat CT imaging that confirms successful conservative management. They should remain on bed rest until their gross hematuria resolves. Discharge criteria are ambulation without recurrence of hematuria, adequate pain control, and toleration of a regular diet. Emphasis should be placed on avoidance of any strenuous activity until follow-up imaging has confirmed resolution of the injury. Grade IV and V renal injuries are serious and the family and the child (if old enough) should be educated about the severity of the injury and the potential signs indicating a delayed complication, such as gross hematuria, worsening abdominal or flank pain,

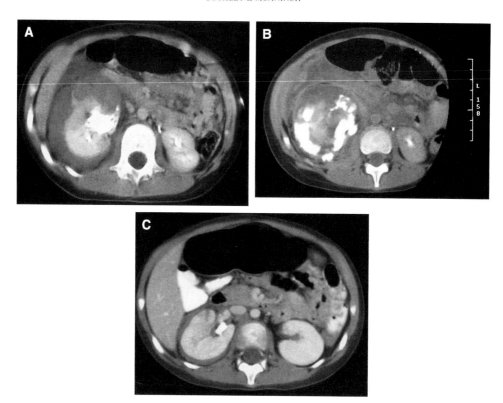

Fig. 3. (A) Diagnostic CT scan at the time of blunt renal trauma with a perirenal hematoma and urinary extravasation. (B) Forty eight–hour interval CT scan showing increased urinary extravasation requiring a ureteral stent. (C) Three-week CT scan showing near complete renal healing with right ureteral stent indwelling.

ileus, or persistent fevers [11]. All severe grade IV to V renal injuries, symptomatic or not, should have postinjury CT or renal isotope imaging at 1 to 3 months to document adequate healing and function [9].

Operative exploration

Operative management still has an important role in the algorithm of pediatric renal trauma. Persistent bleeding is the number one reason for surgical intervention and AAST organ injury severity scale correlates the grade of renal injury with the need for renal exploration and repair [5,9,23,31]. Relative indications for surgical exploration are listed in Box 2 and are assessed on a case-by-case basis. If the patient is being explored for a nonrenal intra-abdominal injury, concomitant renal exploration and reconstruction of any significant renal injury can be performed with excellent renal preservation [9,18,39]. If CT staging or a surgical ICU is not available, renal exploration is favored to ensure a controlled situation and a good outcome.

The recommend operative approach is through a transperitoneal midline incision. The distal aorta is identify and followed cephalad to the left renal vein. If the aorta cannot be identified quickly, the inferior mesenteric vein can be located in the mesentery of the stretched small bowel and the aorta found just medial. The renal vein and artery on the appropriate side are isolated with vessel loops before entering Gerota's fascia for renal

---

Box 2. Indications for renal exploration

Absolute
Expanding renal hematoma
Pulsatile hematoma

Relative
Urinary extravasation
Nonviable tissue
Arterial injury
Incomplete staging

exploration [14,32]. The entire kidney surface is exposed followed by sharp debridement of nonviable tissue, suture ligation of bleeding arterial vessels, and water-tight repair of the collection system. Depending on the type of injury, various reconstruction techniques are applied, such as primary renorrhaphy, omental flap, mesh repair, partial nephrectomy, and vascular repair [14]. Adhering to renal reconstructive techniques preserves renal function and avoids needless nephrectomies [18].

In the AAST organ injury severity scale grade IV to V renal injuries are separated into laceration and vascular injuries [22]. This is an important distinction because the renal salvage rate in vascular injuries, especially main renal artery injuries, is much lower than renal laceration injuries [11,18,40]. Attempted vascular repairs should be limited to minor arterial or venous lacerations or to children with extreme situations, such as a solitary kidney or bilateral renal injuries. Segmental arterial injuries, which are considered a grade IV renal injury, can be managed with observation, angioembolization, or exploration and repair. Observational management is favored and should be followed by selective arterial embolization in the hemodynamically stable child that continues to require blood transfusions.

Outcomes

With renal preservation as the goal, selective operative versus nonoperative management is chosen to achieve optimal success with the least morbidity for the child. Recent large series report a renal salvage rate of >98% in pediatric renal trauma, although follow-up data are limited and incomplete [2,9,21]. In the era of CT imaging, improved critical care units, and growing experience with conservative management, most pediatric renal injuries can be managed nonoperatively with an expected exploration rate between 5% and 11% [20,28]. Although the trend is to manage even the most severe pediatric renal injuries conservatively, judgment should be exercised because some cases are better managed with one definitive surgery rather than delayed interventions that prolong recovery, require additional anesthesia procedures, and ultimately have no renal preservation benefit [41]. Acute complications include persistent or expanding urinomas, expanding hematomas, wound or urinary tract infections, ileus, and pain. Long-term complications include compromised renal function, page kidney causing

hypertension, arteriovenous malformations, and fistula.

Summary

Most pediatric renal trauma is minor and poses no significant danger to the child. A small percentage of children sustain a severe renal injury that demands immediate evaluation and decision of operative versus nonoperative management. Selective management of pediatric renal trauma based on mechanism of injury, hemodynamic stability, associated nonrenal injuries, and CT imaging has led to a renal exploration rate of 5% to 11% with renal salvage rates of >98%.

References

[1] Jacobs IA, Kelly K, Valenziano C, et al. Nonoperative management of blunt splenic and hepatic trauma in the pediatric population: significant differences between adult and pediatric surgeons? Am Surg 2001;67:149.
[2] Nance ML, Lutz N, Carr MC, et al. Blunt renal injuries in children can be managed nonoperatively: outcome in a consecutive series of patients. J Trauma 2004;57:474.
[3] Wessel LM, Scholz S, Jester I, et al. Management of kidney injuries in children with blunt abdominal trauma. J Pediatr Surg 2000;35:1326.
[4] Gerstenbluth RE, Spirnak JP, Elder JS. Sports participation and high grade renal injuries in children. J Urol 2002;168:2575.
[5] Rogers CG, Knight V, MacUra KJ, et al. High-grade renal injuries in children: is conservative management possible? Urology 2004;64:574.
[6] Russell RS, Gomelsky A, McMahon DR, et al. Management of grade IV renal injury in children. J Urol 2001;166:1049.
[7] Kuzmarov IW, Morehouse DD, Gibson S. Blunt renal trauma in the pediatric population: a retrospective study. J Urol 1981;126:648.
[8] Brown SL, Elder JS, Spirnak JP. Are pediatric patients more susceptible to major renal injury from blunt trauma? A comparative study. J Urol 1998;160:138.
[9] Buckley JC, McAninch JW. Pediatric renal injuries: management guidelines from a 25-year experience. J Urol 2004;172:687.
[10] Medica J, Caldamone A. Pediatric renal trauma: special considerations. Semin Urol 1995;13:73.
[11] Santucci RA, Wessells H, Bartsch G, et al. Evaluation and management of renal injuries: consensus statement of the renal trauma subcommittee. BJU Int 2004;93:937.
[12] Armenakas NA, Duckett CP, McAninch JW. Indications for nonoperative management of renal stab wounds. J Urol 1999;161:768.

[13] Livne PM, Gonzales ET Jr. Genitourinary trauma in children. Urol Clin North Am 1985;12:53.

[14] McAninch JW, et al. Renal exploration after trauma: indications and reconstructive techniques. In: Trauma and reconstructive urology. Philadelphia: WB Saunders; 1996. p. 105–12.

[15] Quinlan DM, Gearhart JP. Blunt renal trauma in childhood: features indicating severe injury. Br J Urol 1990;66:526.

[16] Levy JB, Baskin LS, Ewalt DH, et al. Nonoperative management of blunt pediatric major renal trauma. Urology 1993;42:418.

[17] Kansas BT, Eddy MJ, Mydlo JH, et al. Incidence and management of penetrating renal trauma in patients with multiorgan injury: extended experience at an inner city trauma center. J Urol 2004;172:1355.

[18] Wessells H, Deirmenjian J, McAninch JW. Preservation of renal function after reconstruction for trauma: quantitative assessment with radionuclide scintigraphy. J Urol 1997;157:1583.

[19] McAleer IM, Kaplan GW, Scherz HC, et al. Genitourinary trauma in the pediatric patient. Urology 1993;42:563.

[20] Margenthaler JA, Weber TR, Keller MS. Blunt renal trauma in children: experience with conservative management at a pediatric trauma center. J Trauma 2002;52:928.

[21] Radmayr C, Oswald J, Muller E, et al. Blunt renal trauma in children: 26 years clinical experience in an alpine region. Eur Urol 2002;42:297.

[22] Moore EE, Shackford SR, Pachter HL, et al. Organ injury scaling: spleen, liver, and kidney. J Trauma 1989;29:1664.

[23] Smith EM, Elder JS, Spirnak JP. Major blunt renal trauma in the pediatric population: is a nonoperative approach indicated? J Urol 1993;149:546.

[24] Perez-Brayfield MR, Gatti JM, Smith EA, et al. Blunt traumatic hematuria in children: is a simplified algorithm justified? J Urol 2002;167:2543.

[25] Mee SL, McAninch JW. Indications for radiographic assessment in suspected renal trauma. Urol Clin North Am 1989;16:187.

[26] Chandhoke PS, McAninch JW. Detection and significance of microscopic hematuria in patients with blunt renal trauma. J Urol 1988;140:16.

[27] Morey AF, Bruce JE, McAninch JW. Efficacy of radiographic imaging in pediatric blunt renal trauma. J Urol 1996;156:2014.

[28] Nguyen MM, Das S. Pediatric renal trauma. Urology 2002;59:762.

[29] Bretan PN Jr, McAninch JW, Federle MP, et al. Computerized tomographic staging of renal trauma: 85 consecutive cases. J Urol 1986;136:561.

[30] Carpio F, Morey AF. Radiographic staging of renal injuries. World J Urol 1999;17:66.

[31] Santucci RA, McAninch JW, Safir M, et al. Validation of the American Association for the Surgery of Trauma organ injury severity scale for the kidney. J Trauma 2001;50:195.

[32] McAninch JW, Carroll PR. Renal trauma: kidney preservation through improved vascular control-a refined approach. J Trauma 1982;22:285.

[33] Uflacker R, Paolini RM, Lima S. Management of traumatic hematuria by selective renal artery embolization. J Urol 1984;132:662.

[34] Kantor A, Sclafani SJ, Scalea T, et al. The role of interventional radiology in the management of genitourinary trauma. Urol Clin North Am 1989;16: 255.

[35] Wilkinson AG, Haddock G, Carachi R. Separation of renal fragments by a urinoma after renal trauma: percutaneous drainage accelerates healing. Pediatr Radiol 1999;29:503.

[36] Gill B, Palmer LS, Reda E, et al. Optimal renal preservation with timely percutaneous intervention: a changing concept in the management of blunt renal trauma in children in the 1990s. Br J Urol 1994;74: 370.

[37] Philpott JM, Nance ML, Carr MC, et al. Ureteral stenting in the management of urinoma after severe blunt renal trauma in children. J Pediatr Surg 2003; 38:1096.

[38] Moog R, Becmeur F, Dutson E, et al. Functional evaluation by quantitative dimercaptosuccinic acid scintigraphy after kidney trauma in children. J Urol 2003;169:641.

[39] Angus LD, Tachmes L, Kahn S, et al. Surgical management of pediatric renal trauma: an urban experience. Am Surg 1993;59:388.

[40] Knudson MM, Harrison PB, Hoyt DB, et al. Outcome after major renovascular injuries: a Western trauma association multicenter report. J Trauma 2000;49:1116.

[41] Delarue A, Merrot T, Fahkro A, et al. Major renal injuries in children: the real incidence of kidney loss. J Pediatr Surg 2002;37:1446.

ELSEVIER
SAUNDERS

Urol Clin N Am 33 (2006) 41–53

UROLOGIC
CLINICS
of North America

Complications of Renal Trauma

Hosam S. Al-Qudah, MD[a], Richard A. Santucci, MD[a,b],*

[a]Department of Urology, Wayne State University School of Medicine
[b]Detroit Receiving Hospital, 4160 John R. Suite 1017, Detroit, MI 48201, USA

Renal trauma occurs in 1% to 3% of all trauma cases [1]. Complications after renal trauma occur between 3% and 33% of these patients [2–4]. A wide range of reported complications exists in those with renal trauma. In 2001, Blankenship and colleagues [3] reported that one third of conservatively treated renal trauma patients develop one or more urologic complications, whereas other series have had much lower complication rates closer to 5% [5,6]. Complications of renal trauma have been reviewed in the past, in 1989 and 2001 [4,7], and this review is intended to update and widen these older reports.

Extravasation of urine

Extravasation of urine is the most common complication of renal trauma [8] and is present in all patients, by definition, with stage IV parenchymal renal trauma and also may be caused by forniceal rupture after lesser trauma [9]. The prevalence of extravasation is higher after penetrating injury (10%–30%) than after blunt trauma (2%–18%) [7,10]. In rare cases, urinary extravasation may result from direct trauma to the renal pelvis or ureteropelvic junction (UPJ) injury [11–13].

Diagnosis and treatment

The sensitivity of intravenous pyelogram (IVP) the diagnosis of urinary extravasation after renal trauma and leak is about 70% [14–16]. In most centers, computed tomography (CT) scan has replaced IVP and has a higher diagnostic accuracy

for urine leak [1,7,17,18]. The preferred CT protocol in many trauma centers is a helical scan of the abdomen and pelvis, with an early arterial and/or venous portal phase, and a late 10-minute delayed images to detect urine leakage [1]. Some specific findings on CT can be particularly helpful. For example, medial extravasation of the contrast and absence of ureteral opacification is diagnostic of renal pelvis injury and typically is seen without perinephric hematoma [11]. A lack of ureteral filling differentiates between UPJ avulsion (no ureteral filling seen) and medial renal or renal pelvis laceration [19]. Diagnosis of this serious entity is delayed in more than 50% of cases [12,13], and scrupulous use of delayed CT films in CT scan decreases the number of missed injuries in these patients [13,20].

In only 13% to 26% of cases urinary leakage persists for longer than a few days of expectant management, which includes bed rest, antimicrobials, and analgesics without antiplatelet effects [8,21,22]. Conservative treatment does not seem to increase hospital stay or compromise outcomes [4,21,23,24]. Even extensive extravasation is likely to subside without intervention. The authors tend to advocate the use of antimicrobials in patients who present with active urinary extravasation or large perirenal hematoma (especially if they have open wounds as with road burn), although no randomized clinical trials exist that absolutely support their use.

Monitoring with serial CT scans is controversial. The authors use CT scans aggressively in cases of fever, dropping hematocrit, persistent flank pain, or other symptoms that might indicate complications surrounding the injured kidney. A single follow-up CT scan may be valuable to document the resolution of extravasation or the development of occult complications [25].

* Corresponding author. Detroit Receiving Hospital, 4160 John R. Suite 1017, Detroit, MI 48201.
E-mail address: rsantucc@med.wayne.edu (R.A. Santucci).

In those rare cases whereby extravasation persists unduly, or is complicated by enlarging urinoma or urine leakage from a surgical wound, most patients are cured durably by the placement of a ureteral stent retrograde by way of cystoscopy or anterograde after percutaneous nephrostomy [8,24,26–28]. One case in which urinary extravasation may be more complicated is in the presence of devascularized segment, which may increase the chance of urinoma or abscess. Although Husmann and Morris reported a complication rate of 38% in these patients when treated conservatively [29], others have not been able to reproduce these findings [30]. This risk for complications also may be increased in those patients who present with associated pancreatic, colonic, or major soft tissue trauma [18,21,29]. Exploration and repair of at least the colon or pancreatic injury is advisable in these patients, with the consideration of colostomy for patients who present with colonic trauma [31]. The surgical field should be well drained after exploration [18].

Urinoma

Urinoma is a urine collection that may form after trauma when urine extravasates through major parenchymal disruptions or UPJ laceration. Urinoma may be worsened in cases of distal urinary obstruction [7,32,33]. Urinoma may be seen in 1% to 7% of renal trauma patients [7,34,35]. Urinoma may be seen more commonly in patients who present with penetrating trauma (7%–30%) [10,34].

Presentation and diagnosis

Urinoma is often asymptomatic and may be suspected in patients who present with abdominal pain, low grade fever, ileus, or a palpable mass [7,36]. CT scan is the preferred modality of evaluation. Most urinoma is acute, but in rare cases it can present from 3 weeks to several years after injury [4,7,37].

Urinoma may appear on CT scan as confined or free fluid in the intra or retroperitoneal compartments [13]. Most urinomas are found in a subcapsular location or in the perirenal space within the Gerota's fascia [38]. When especially large, urinoma may extend medially, even crossing the aorta and inferior vena cava. Commonly, it can extend inferiorly along the iliopsoas compartment into the pelvis, and rarely may even track into the soft tissue of the thigh, pelvis, buttocks,

scrotum, or perineum. Superior extension through diaphragm to the plural space or through the aortic hiatus into the mediastinum has been reported [33,39–42].

On CT, urinoma has an attenuation range from 0 to 20 Housfield Units (HU) before intravenous contrast injection and may enhance up to 200 HU after contrast administration. Caution is warranted as normal ascites fluid may enhance on delayed contrast CT studies up to 54 HU in the absence of bleeding, bowel perforation, or urinary leakage, and care must be taken not to mistake ascites for urinoma in these cases [43]. After time, a fibrous capsule surrounding the urinoma may be present, and it may calcify rarely [44]. Although some centers, especially in Europe, advocate ultrasound for the diagnosis and follow-up of urinoma, the authors believe CT scan has distinct advantages over ultrasound for showing kidney function, active urine leak, improved anatomic delineation, and better evaluation of other organ injury [7]. Some have suggested that renal scintigraphy be used as an alternative to CT scan in patients who present with impaired renal function or contrast allergy, although it is likely that this modality will rarely be used at most centers [33].

Treatment

Most urinomas are absorbed and there is no need to intervene [7,33]; however, radiologic re-evaluation should be done to exclude continuous leak, increase in size, or persistence [7,25]. Indications for intervention mostly are relative and include huge urinoma; persistent urinoma (although no absolute cutoff point exists and most observe urinomas, especially if not growing, for several days); development of fever or sepsis; and urinoma that separates renal fragments (some experts believe that treating the urinoma improves acceleration of healing and preservation of renal function) [33,45].

No best way exists to treat all patients who present with urinoma. The authors recommend maximizing draining by placing a retrograde stent, whereas others describe starting with percutaneous drainage of the urinoma alone [33]. If percutaneous drainage is used, simultaneous stent or percutaneous nephrostomy is prudent. Ureteral stents have distinct advantages over percutaneous drains by the avoidance of catheter care, avoiding urine bags, and absence of dislodgment potential [27]. In modern series, anterograde stents without percutaneous nephrostomy are possible in the majority (90%–100%) of patients [26]. Ureteral stent placement is *not* recommended in cases of renal pelvis laceration, which likely will need open repair [7]. If retrograde stenting is not possible technically, percutaneous drainage is an excellent technique [46]. Neither technique seems more advantageous than the other in efficacy of urinary drainage [27].

In rare, extreme cases, other therapies may be tried. Some have reported using selective embolization of the renal parenchyma, which reduces the urine filling a refractory urinoma as an alternative to open surgery [28,47]. Surgery can be used, although rarely in cases refractory to more conservative treatment [4].

Perinephric abscess

Urinary tract infection is one of the main infections reported in all trauma patients in the intensive care unit [48]. In rare cases, urinary infections can be symptomatic of a more serious infection—a perinephric abscess. The preferred examination in suspected cases is CT scan [7].

Perinephric abscess is rare, and in a series of 25 patients only 4 had a traumatic etiology for the abscess [49]. Frank abscess occurs in less than 1% of renal trauma cases, [2,10] and in 5% of penetrating renal trauma cases. [16]. An interesting series showed that 5% of conservatively treated patients developed abscess compared with 2% of surgically treated renal injuries [16]; however, other series have not seen these negative results from nonoperative treatment of renal trauma [5]. Husmann and colleagues [29] reported increased infectious complications in 11 patients who presented with devascularized segments after renal trauma. Four out of 11 patients (26%) developed perinephric abscess and 3 out of 11 (27%) developed an infected urinoma. All abscesses occurred in patients with bowel or pancreatic laceration or large areas of soft tissue loss requiring debridement [29].

Abscess should be suspected in patients who present with fever after urinoma or perinephric hematoma and may be more common in those with predisposing factors, such as devitalized segment, coexisting enteric or pancreatic injury, devitalized colonic or duodenal injuries, infected central line, large areas of soft tissue loss requiring debridement, diabetes, HIV, or drug abuse [21,29,50–52]. An elevated serum neutrophil count, flank tenderness, and persistent ileus also can be present. Infectious complications usually occur 5 to 7 days after renal injury [7]. Chronic abscess present as persistent lethargy, night sweats, anorexia, and unexplained weight loss [7].

CT scan is the modality of choice for evaluation of suspected abscess. Abscesses appear as 10 to 60 HU fluid collection with or without loculations. Gas pockets may be present [7]. The high mortality of perinephric abscess (12%–57%) usually is caused by delay in diagnosis [49,53]. Death is uncommon with early diagnosis [49]. Treatment may start with antibiotics alone when it is less than 3 cm. Larger abscesses need percutaneous catheter drainage in addition to antibiotics. Repeated imaging is mandatory to evaluate resolution, and nephrectomy should be performed in a poorly functioning kidney with persistent infection [49,53].

Coincident organ injury

The presence of coincident organ injury is not a complication itself, but it is a complicating factor of renal trauma. Associated organ injury is reported in 61% to 100% of reported cases of penetrating renal trauma [10,51,54,55], and 35% to 65% of reported blunt renal trauma cases [6,8,56].

Hepatic injury is seen commonly in those with renal injury and may be seen in 73% of right penetrating renal trauma and 30% of blunt renal trauma [57]. Associated hepatic injury occurs in 26% to 33% of penetrating renal trauma [51,55], whereas splenic injury is reported in 22% to 39% of penetrating renal trauma [51,55].

Associated pancreatic injury is much more rare, occurring in only 1.6% of blunt kidney trauma patients in general. Penetrating trauma may be associated with pancreatic injury in higher rates, from 15% to 26%. [51,55]. Older reports showed that pancreatic injury is associated with higher complication rates, especially fistula and perinephric abscess. These complications were so serious that in 1976, Radwin and colleagues [58] went as far as to recommend nephrectomy to all patients who presented with associated pancreatic injury. In more modern series, greatly increased complications were not seen in coincident renal and pancreatic injury, and nephrectomy is recommended only for patients who present with such severe renal injury that repair is impossible [52]. Pancreatic injuries, however, may herald a high 15% complication rate [52].

Colonic injury and small bowel injury is reported after penetrating renal trauma in 38% to 48% of patients [51,55]; however, only colonic injury increases the risk for complications (perinephric abscess) [51].

Unnecessary nephrectomy

Although not classically considered a "complication," the authors consider the unnecessary removal of a kidney during the treatment of renal trauma to be an avoidable disaster second only to death or extreme debility. Although this problem occurs less frequently now that conservative management of renal trauma is more common, between 17% and 30% of traumatized kidneys were spared nephrectomy when conservative therapy became hospital policy [6,24,59,60]. For patients who require exploration and nephrectomy, data suggest that nephrectomy rates also can be decreased by using early vascular control, which alone decreased nephrectomy rate from 56% to 18% in one important series [61]. Although authors have written that trauma nephrectomy is seldom a direct cause of death (except in patients who present with renal pedicle injury and attendant massive bleeding) [17], the authors believe that the severely injured patient is most in need of maximum kidney function. The cost of losing a kidney is not zero. In one small series, 28% of post trauma nephrectomy patients had renal failure, and this was believed to increase mortality in a subset of patients [62].

Even the risk for unnecessary surgical exploration might be considered a "complication" of renal injury management [4]. Unnecessary exploration used to be common, in the 37% to 39% range, in cases of penetrating renal trauma [63,64] but is much less common now that CT is used frequently and conservative therapy often attempted.

Impaired kidney function and renal insufficiency

Preservation of renal function while minimizing morbidity and eliminating renal-related mortality is the authors' goal when treating renal trauma patients. According to the literature, often this is possible. Wessells and colleagues [65] reported that renal function by radionuclide scan was 39% after renal reconstruction in 52 patients. Nineteen percent of patients had less than 33% function in the injured side, and only one patient had renal insufficiency requiring dialysis (bilateral

kidney injury, one side nephrectomy, and the other renorrhaphy). El-Sherbiny and colleages [66] recently reported no cases of renal insufficiency in 13 children with high-grade renal trauma whom were treated conservatively despite morphologic change in 92% of them. A more recent report showed that renal function was preserved in children with Grade II-IV injury after conservative treatment, but that those with Grade V injures had a mean of 29% function [67]. In general, good results after expert care for renal injury has been documented in 93% to 100% of kidney trauma patients [24,68–70]. Not surprisingly, those patients that require nephrectomy for trauma have the worse kidney function compared with patients who have renorrhaphy or conservative treatment [71]. Acute renal failure can be multifactorial in ill trauma patients, but one series found that renal failure was seen in 6% of penetrating renal trauma patients [72].

Hypertension

Development of hypertension after renal trauma is a controversial issue. Although its occurrence has been widely reported, many series have not observed it [10,20,51,54,56,59,70,73]. In general, it may occur an average in 5% of renal trauma patients [74]. Reports range widely from 0.2% to 55% [2,24,75–79]. In one study, the prevalence of hypertension in conservatively treated patients was 55% compared with 0% in surgically treated patients [78]; however, these high rates of post injury hypertension have not been repeated in multiple other reports [2,74,75,79]. Dobrowolski and colleagues [2] reported identical rates of hypertension in surgically or conservatively treated renal trauma patients. Transient hypertension is sometimes seen after injury, occurring in 6% to 10% of patients with renal trauma [59,80]. This temporary condition reverted to normal in 12 to 50 days. Chronic hypertension after renal trauma develops in a period ranging from 2 days to 32 years [74,81,82].

Hypertension can be caused by three mechanisms. First, injury to the renal artery or one of its branches causes arterial stenosis or occlusion (Goldblatt kidney) [82,83]. Second, increased pressure on the kidney acutely from hematoma (often subcapsular hematoma) or chronically from scar decreases renal blood flow, the "so-called" Page kidney. Third, traumatic arterio-venous fistula can result in renal hemodynamic changes. [73]. All three mechanisms are similar in that they lead to reduction in renal blood flow, which stimulates the kidney to produce renin [1,84].

The incidence of post-traumatic hypertension is affected by the severity of renal trauma and the prevalence of preexisting essential hypertension, which itself is affected by the age, sex, and race of the population [1]. Danuser and colleagues [59] reviewed 62 patients after renal trauma with a mean follow-up of 13 years and found that 10% developed permanent hypertension in 4 to 12 years after trauma. This was *not* elevated compared with the 12% rate of hypertension in age equivalent control groups. Several other reports exist that also did not show any renovascular hypertension after renal trauma [10,20,51,54,56,70,73]. An excellent report by Monstrey and colleagues [85] retrospectively reviewed 435 kidney trauma patients and performed literature analysis of another 223 cases of post-traumatic hypertension. The report concluded that renal trauma could not be linked to an increased incidence of hypertension and criticized the widespread acceptance of cause-effect when hypertension is incidentally found in a patient who at some point had renal trauma [85].

One well-documented source of post-injury hypertension is renal artery occlusion, which, although rare, may cause hypertension in a significant percentage (32%–50%) of patients in whom it is present [6,86,87]. One series reporting the rate of hypertension to be as high as 42% in conservatively treated patients who presented with known renal artery occlusion, which fell to 3% with surgical treatment [88].

Diagnosis

A high index of suspension is the key factor for diagnosis of renovascular hypertension in trauma patients, most of whom are young and without co-morbidities. Patients can present with unusual symptoms, such as hypertensive encephalopathy, nose bleed, chest pain, or myocardial infarction [74]. The gold standard for the diagnosis of post-traumatic renovascular hypertension is selective angiography and renal vein renin measurements. Elevated renin from the diseased kidney in a ratio of less than 1.5:1 compared with the other side predicts response to surgical treatment in more than 90% of cases [84,89].

Treatment

As spontaneous resolution has been reported in multiple studies, it is always advisable to start with conservative treatment. Hypertension that is well controlled temporarily by one or two medications will save the patient a major vascular surgery or partial or total nephrectomy if the condition resolves with time. Conservative therapy was effective in two out seven (28%) patients in one study and two out of five (40%) in another [81,84]. Surgery, including renal revascularization, partial nephrectomy or even total nephrectomy is the second step of management. In cases of total arterial obstruction, Watts reported that nephrectomy performed within the first year of injury had better response rates (96% compared with 60%) [74]. Response rates to nephrectomy ranged from 88% to 100% in different series [76,82,84].

Page kidney

The first report of renin dependent hypertension was published by Page in 1939 [90]. Hypertension was induced by experimentally wrapping a canine kidney with cellophane. Page described formation of thick, dense, scar tissue around the kidney producing constrictive perinephritis and hypertension. The blood pressure returned to normal after nephrectomy. In 1955, Engel and Page reported the first clinical correlation with this experiment in a 19-year-old hypertensive man cured by removal of the kidney that was compressed by an old calcified subcapsular hematoma [91]. After that report hypertension secondary to renal compression was referred to as "Page kidney."

Pathophysiology

Because Page first described the disease there had been many case reports [92]. The cause of the renal compression varied, including hematoma secondary to blunt trauma, renal biopsy, anticoagulation, vasculitis, tumor hemorrhage, extracorporeal shock wave lithotripsy, sympathetic nerve block, and pyeloplasty [93–98]. For patients without hematoma, Page kidney is reportedly caused by urinoma [99,100], renal cyst [101], pararenal lymphocele [102], perirenal pseudocyst [103], and retroperitoneal paraganglioma [104].

External compression of the kidney causes renal hypoperfusion and ischemia that activates the renin-angiotensin-aldosterone axis resulting in salt and water retention and hypertension [90,92,93,101]. This compression may be caused by the perirenal collection itself and may explain cases with the early presentations after trauma that disappears within one month, after resolution of hematoma, or by percutaneous management of the collection. The compression also may be caused by extensive scaring caused by the extrarenal hematoma or from scarring of the renal capsule [7]. Theoretically, only a few millimeters of capsular thickening or contraction are needed to cause renal compression.

Diagnosis and treatment

The most common presentation of post-traumatic Page kidney is in an otherwise healthy adult with a new onset of hypertension and a history of renal trauma that may be new or remote. CT is the preferred modality of initial evaluation. In early cases, CT may demonstrate subcapsular hematoma, appearing as a rounded area of low attenuation located between the renal cortex and the capsule, which is indenting the renal parenchyma [105]. Late cases show attenuated contrast enhancement of the kidney, with a fibrotic band surrounding the kidney, which may be calcified [7,106].

In acute cases, MRI may have the advantage of allowing estimation of the age of the hematoma, which may have therapeutic implication. Arteriography shows a diffusely enlarged kidney with delayed contrast perfusion on the affected side with stretching of the segmental and interpolar arteries [7].

The aim of treatment is to cure the hypertension and preserve the kidney [92]. In acute cases, therapy starts with angiotensin converting enzyme inhibitors to control the blood pressure while waiting for local hematoma to be absorbed. Large liquid hematomas may respond to percutaneous drainage. Patients who present with old hematoma, or severely impaired kidney function, may need active intervention including capsulectomy, partial nephrectomy (if compression is to a polar area), or a total nephrectomy [7,92,107]. Watts and colleagues [74] reported in a review paper that nephrectomy cured hypertension in 89% of 18 patients. Although technically challenging, Page kidney has been treated laparoscopically with dissection of the perinephric fibrosis [107].

Specific complications of renal vascular injury

Of all the types of renal injury, renal vascular injury is the most dangerous. These injuries occur in 2.5% to 4% of renal trauma patients and in 16% of patients who present with penetrating abdominal injuries [1]. They usually occur in significantly injured patients and are associated with much higher risk for morbidity (transfusion rate, impaired kidney function, nephrectomy, and other complications) and mortality [7,108]. Associated injuries occurs in most (72%–100%) [1,86,108,109]. In a review of several large series, the nephrectomy rate after renovascular injury was 6 to 12 fold higher than after renal parenchymal injury (nephrectomy rate of 30%–60% compared with 5% in parenchymal trauma) [7]. Mortality was likewise high in the renovascular group, ranging between 19% and 44% [1]. The chance that nephrectomy will be required is also high, ranging from 67% to 78% after arterial injury and 71% to 74% after arterial thrombosis [1]. Isolated renal vein injury is rare but, when present, has a higher chance of successful repair except for avulsion from inferior vena cava in which nephrectomy is usually required immediately [1,110,111].

Renal trauma and congenital anomalies

The reported incidence of congenital anomalies of the kidney in renal trauma varies in different series from 1% to 23% [4,112,113]. Preexisting congenital renal abnormalities seem to increase the risk for significant renal injury and to decrease the potential for renal salvage [114,115]. For example, UPJ stenosis was believed to increase the chance of renal pelvic avulsion after renal trauma and to lower the threshold for renal bleeding following minor trauma [4,57]. Significant preexisting UPJ obstruction may limit the leakage of renal blood into the bladder and, thus, may cause absence of hematuria in a high percentage of patients who present with renal trauma (31%) [116].

Some series suggest that the presence of congenital anomalies does not increase the morbidity or mortality of renal trauma patients [117]. The conventional wisdom, however, is that congenital abnormalities not only predispose to injury (they were present in 36% of children who presented with renal trauma in one series) but causes more post-injury complications compared with children without preexisting kidney lesions [118].

Secondary hemorrhage

Secondary hemorrhage is one of the most serious complications of renal trauma. It is more common in cases of deep cortical lacerations, especially in stab wounds patients treated conservatively [7,64]. Some series have reported delayed bleeding in 13% to 25% of grade 3–4 blunt renal trauma patients who are treated conservatively

[34] and in 18% to 23% of penetrating renal trauma patients who are treated conservatively [7,54,119, 120]. It must be noted, however, that a bleeding rate of 0% is seen in several similar reports [5]. Delayed hematuria can occur in 3% to 15% of patients following primary surgical exploration after renal trauma [111,120,121]. Most cases of delayed bleeding are believed to be caused by a traumatic pseudoaneurysm or arteriovenous fistula (AVF) (Fig. 1) [120]. Other bleeds may be caused by segmental renal artery bleeding. Acutely, this bleeding usually is stopped by tamponade of hematoma formation, but after hematoma resolution (hematoma liquefaction takes 5–14 days) the artery may rebleed [1,18]. Bleeding may be into the collecting system or into the perirenal space and may be life-threatening [122]. Timing for this bleeding most commonly is in the first 2 to 3 weeks of renal trauma (range from 2–45 days) [1,64,123]. A reported case of pseudoaneurysm occurs 15 years after conservative management of penetrating renal trauma [124].

Arteriovenous fistula

AVF is, most commonly, a result of renal biopsy [7,125], but post-traumatic AVF rarely occurs, mostly in stab wound patients [126]. Reports of AVF complicating stab wounds ranged from 0% to 7% [10,54,126]. Watts and colleagues [74] reported 12 cases of AVF in a review paper of hypertension, 10 of them caused by penetrating trauma and two by blunt trauma. Unlike postbiopsy AVF, which resolve spontaneously in 50% to 70% of cases, post-traumatic AVF often need intervention, such as percutaneous ablation by interventional radiology [1]. Rarely, urgent nephrectomy is needed.

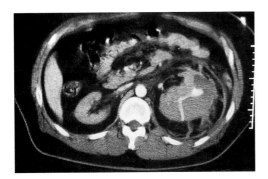

Fig. 1. Arterial-venous malformation with connection to renal pelvis after renal stab wound, resulting in massive hematuria.

Diagnosis and treatment

Clinical manifestation of AVF depends on size and location. It causes urinary problems presenting as hematuria (microscopic or macroscopic) with or without clot retention and cardiovascular problems, including diastolic hypertension, cardiomegaly, and congestive heart failure [125]. AVF is sometimes detectable by physical examination by the presence of an abdominal bruit. Suspected AVF likely requires angiography [7], with planned simultaneous embolization, although renal scintigraphy has been said to be diagnostic in some cases [1,18]. Magnetic resonance angiography (MRA) can be used in patients who present with contrast allergy or impaired renal function. Ishikawa recently reported two cases of arteriovenous fistula that CT failed to diagnose and were diagnosed by MRA [127]. Small AVF that cause microscopic hematuria usually do not require treatment [126]. Superselective embolization is generally a safe and effective treatment modality for AVF with minimal associated morbidity [128–130]. Rare complications of embolization do occur, including abscess, postembolization syndrome, segmental infarction, impaired renal function, pulmonary embolization of coils, allergic reaction, and nonexpanding hematoma at arterial puncture site [131–134].

Pseudoaneurysm

Pseudoaneurysm is a well-reported complication after parenchymal renal surgery [123]. Pseudoaneurysm is reported after percutaneous surgery, open surgery, renal biopsy, and endoscopic renal surgery [135]. Penetrating renal trauma is the second most common cause (after iatrogenic) and occurred in 6% of 93 patients after renal stab wounds [120]. Pseudoaneurysm also is described in several cases after blunt renal trauma [123,136–140]. Pseudoaneurysm can grow over time, sometimes becoming unstable and eroding into the surrounding pelvicaleceal system or surrounding perinephric tissue [123,141]. Pseudoaneurysm usually presents with one or more of the following symptoms: gross hematuria, flank pain, mass, abdominal bruit, or hypertension [123].

Diagnosis and treatment

Doppler ultrasound can be useful in the diagnosis of pseudoaneurysm, although CT is likely the initial study of choice. On ultrasound, the lesion appears as an anechoic lesion and with Doppler enhancement may have a characteristic to-and-fro swirling [105,123].

In one small study CT was diagnostic in three out of three patients [123]. A scanning technique using thin cuts of the renal fossa is recommended by experts. Pseudoaneurysm usually enhances in the arterial phase and washes out in the delayed phase [105,123].

Angiography is the gold standard for evaluation of pseudoaneurysm and is usually performed only after Doppler ultrasound or CT scan, although there are reported cases that were missed with both modalities [138,142]. Pseudoaneurysms appears as round or oval structures that opacify from the main renal artery or from one of its branches [143].

Embolization is the first line of treatment. Although rare, the most common complication after embolization is the postembolization syndrome subsequent to inadvertent large volume parenchymal infarction [144]. Modern "superselective" embolization techniques should decrease the incidence of this problem [131,145]. Chatziioannou and colleagues [146] recently reported in a small series of angioembolization with a mean of 12% loss of parenchyma immediately after embolization which decreased to 6% on follow-up CT scan.

Death

Mortality after renal trauma is influenced by several factors, including the nature of the trauma, quality and timing of resuscitation, associated injuries, and subsequent complications [4]. Mortality in patients who present with renal trauma is almost always a result of associated injuries, and mortality from renal trauma accounts for less than 0.1% of trauma deaths [7]. As expected, penetrating trauma has higher mortality rates than blunt trauma, ranging from 6% to 8% [51,72]. Among patients who expired after trauma nephrectomy, those who died had significantly lower systolic blood pressures, higher injury severity score, higher incidence of extra-abdominal injuries, shorter operative times, and higher estimated blood loss. The investigators concluded that nephrectomy is usually done in severely injured unstable patients and mortality is secondary to the severity of the overall constellation of injury and is not a consequence of nephrectomy itself [147].

Miscellaneous complications

Postinjury hydronephrosis

Hydronephrosis after renal injury is reported in 0% to 3% of cases [78]. Some investigators have suggested that new hydronephrosis after injury is more common after conservative therapy than surgical therapy. Cass and colleagues [78] reported 62% of conservatively treated patients compared with 4% of surgically treated patients developed hydronephrosis. The etiology of new hydronephrosis after injury is not understood well. It may be caused by UPJ obstruction from perirenal and periureteral fibrosis [7], perhaps caused by urine extravasation, hematoma, abscess, or pyelonephritis. Patients may be symptomatic or asymptomatic and may present with flank pain depending on the speed of obstruction development. Management of hydronephrosis depends on the degree of obstruction and its effect on kidney function. In symptomatic, obstructed cases treatment may include pyeloplasty or even nephrectomy in poorly functioning kidneys.

Flank pain

It is reported that after renal trauma 2% to 12% of patients complain of ipsilateral flank pain [77,79]. This pain can be a result of UPJ obstruction, perinephric abscess, or persistent urinoma, and treatment depends on etiology. CT scan with delayed images, followed by directed studies (such as lasix renogram in cases of suspected UPJ obstruction), are warranted.

Fistula

Renocutaneos fistula is a rare complication after renal trauma. In one series, it was reported in 15% of patient after surgical repair of the kidney, including partial nephrectomy, renorrhaphy, or open drainage of collection but in general is seldom seen or reported [24]. Ureteral catheter placement is the treatment of choice [24].

Pulmonary complications

Pulmonary complications are common in all trauma patients [72,148], and include pneumonia, bronchitis, atelectasis, and iatrogenic pnemothorax. Pulmonary complications may be more common for patients who require surgical management of renal trauma. Pulmonary complications occurred in 4% of those with conservatively treated stab wound patients but in 33% to 38% of surgically treated stab wounds in one series [121]. Pulmonary complications occurred in 12% of patients after gun shot renal trauma [149].

Other

Chylous ascitis has been reported after trauma nephrectomy in a single patient [150].

References

[1] Santucci RA, Wessells H, Bartsch G, et al. Evaluation and management of renal injuries: consensus statement of the renal trauma subcommittee. BJU Int 2004;93:937–54.

[2] Dobrowolski Z, Kusionowicz J, Drewniak T, et al. Renal and ureteric trauma: diagnosis and management in Poland. BJU Int 2002;89:748–51.

[3] Blankenship JC, Gavant ML, Cox CE, et al. Importance of delayed imaging for blunt renal trauma. World J Surg 2001;25:1561–4.

[4] Peterson NE. Complications of renal trauma. Urol Clin North Am 1989;16:221–36.

[5] Hammer CC, Santucci RA. Effect of an institutional policy of nonoperative treatment of grades I to IV renal injuries. J Urol 2003;169:1751–3.

[6] Goff CD, Collin GR. Management of renal trauma at a rural, level I trauma center. Am Surg 1998;64:226–30.

[7] Brandes SB, McAninch JW. Complications of renal trauma. In: Taneja SS, Smith RB, Ehrlich RM, editors. Complications of urology. 3rd edition. Philadelphia: W.B. Saunders; 2001. p. 205–25.

[8] Matthews LA, Smith EM, Spirnak JP. Nonoperative treatment of major blunt renal lacerations with urinary extravasation. J Urol 1997;157:2056–8.

[9] Brandes SB, McAninch JW. Reconstructive surgery for trauma of the upper urinary tract. Urol Clin North Am 1999;26:183–99.

[10] Kansas BT, Eddy MJ, Mydlo JH, et al. Incidence and management of penetrating renal trauma in patients with multiorgan injury: extended experience at an inner city trauma center. J Urol 2004;172:1355–60.

[11] Kawashima A, Sandler CM, Corl FM, et al. Imaging of renal trauma: a comprehensive review. Radiographics 2001;21:557–74.

[12] Boone TB, Gilling PJ, Husmann DA. Ureteropelvic junction disruption following blunt abdominal trauma. J Urol 1993;150:33–6.

[13] Mulligan JM, Cagiannos I, Collins JP, et al. Ureteropelvic junction disruption secondary to blunt trauma: excretory phase imaging (delayed films) should help prevent a missed diagnosis. J Urol 1998;159:67–70.

[14] Thall EH, Stone NN, Cheng DL, et al. Conservative management of penetrating and blunt Type III renal injuries. Br J Urol 1996;77:512–7.

[15] Erturk E, Sheinfeld J, DiMarco PL, et al. Renal trauma: evaluation by computerized tomography. J Urol 1985;133:946–9.

[16] Wilson RF, Ziegler DW. Diagnostic and treatment problems in renal injuries. Am Surg 1987;53:399–402.

[17] Cass AS, Cerra FB, Luxenberg M, et al. Renal failure and mortality after nephrectomy for severe trauma in multiply-injured patient: no inordinate risk. Urology 1987;30:213–5.

[18] Heyns CF. Renal trauma: indications for imaging and surgical exploration. BJU Int 2004;93:1165–70.

[19] Kawashima A, Sandler CM, Corriere JN Jr, et al. Ureteropelvic junction injuries secondary to blunt abdominal trauma. Radiology 1997;205:487–92.

[20] Nance ML, Lutz N, Carr MC, et al. Blunt renal injuries in children can be managed nonoperatively: outcome in a consecutive series of patients. J Trauma 2004;57:474–8 [discussion: 478].

[21] Moudouni SM, Patard JJ, Manunta A, et al. A conservative approach to major blunt renal lacerations with urinary extravasation and devitalized renal segments. BJU Int 2001;87:290–4.

[22] Rogers CG, Knight V, MacUra KJ, et al. High-grade renal injuries in children–is conservative management possible? Urology 2004;64:574–9.

[23] Matthews LA, Spirnak JP. The nonoperative approach to major blunt renal trauma. Semin Urol 1995;13:77–82.

[24] Moudouni SM, Hadj Slimen M, Manunta A, et al. Management of major blunt renal lacerations: is a nonoperative approach indicated? Eur Urol 2001;40:409–14.

[25] Meng MV, Brandes SB, McAninch JW. Renal trauma: indications and techniques for surgical exploration. World J Urol 1999;17:71–7.

[26] Haas CA, Reigle MD, Selzman AA, et al. Use of ureteral stents in the management of major renal trauma with urinary extravasation: is there a role? J Endourol 1998;12:545–9.

[27] Philpott JM, Nance ML, Carr MC, et al. Ureteral stenting in the management of urinoma after severe blunt renal trauma in children. J Pediatr Surg 2003;38:1096–8.

[28] Horikami K, Matsuoka Y, Nagaoki K, et al. Treatment of post-traumatic urinoma by means of selective arterial embolization. J Vasc Interv Radiol 1997;8:221–4.

[29] Husmann DA, Morris JS. Attempted nonoperative management of blunt renal lacerations extending through the corticomedullary junction: the short-term and long-term sequelae. J Urol 1990;143:682–4.

[30] Peterson NE. Fate of functionless post-traumatic renal segment. Urology 1986;27:237–42.

[31] Wessells H, McAninch JW. Effect of colon injury on the management of simultaneous renal trauma. J Urol 1996;155:1852–6.

[32] McInerney D, Jones A, Roylance J. Urinoma. Clin Radiol 1977;28:345–51.

[33] Titton RL, Gervais DA, Hahn PF, et al. Urine leaks and urinomas: diagnosis and imaging-guided intervention. Radiographics 2003;23:1133–47.

[34] Gibson S, Kuzmarov IW, McClure DR, et al. Blunt renal trauma: the value of a conservative approach to major injuries in clinically stable patients. Can J Surg 1982;25:25–6.

[35] Mansi MK, Alkhudair WK. Conservative management with percutaneous intervention of major blunt renal injuries. Am J Emerg Med 1997;15: 633–7.

[36] Morano JU, Burkhalter JL. Percutaneous catheter drainage of post-traumatic urinoma. J Urol 1985; 134:319–21.

[37] Thompson IM, Latourette H, Montie JE, et al. Results of non-operative management of blunt renal trauma. Trans Am Assoc Genitourin Surg 1976;68:128–31.

[38] Gore RM, Balfe DM, Aizenstein RI, et al. The great escape: interfascial decompression planes of the retroperitoneum. Am J Roentgenol 2000;175: 363–70.

[39] Lang EK, Glorioso L III. Management of urinomas by percutaneous drainage procedures. Radiol Clin North Am 1986;24:551–9.

[40] Oguzulgen IK, Oguzulgen AI, Sinik Z, et al. An unusual cause of urinothorax. Respiration (Herrlisheim) 2002;69:273–4.

[41] Lahiry SK, Alkhafaji AH, Brown AL. Urinothorax following blunt trauma to the kidney. J Trauma 1978;18:608–10.

[42] Parvathy U, Saldanha R, Balakrishnan KR. Blunt abdominal trauma resulting in urinothorax from a missed uretero-pelvic junction avulsion: case report. J Trauma 2003;54:187–9.

[43] Cooper C, Silverman PM, Davros WJ, et al. Delayed contrast enhancement of ascitic fluid on CT: frequency and significance. Am J Roentgenol 1993;161:787–90.

[44] Gayer G, Zissin R, Apter S, et al. Urinomas caused by ureteral injuries: CT appearance. Abdom Imaging 2002;27:88–92.

[45] Wilkinson AG, Haddock G, Carachi R. Separation of renal fragments by a urinoma after renal trauma: percutaneous drainage accelerates healing. Pediatr Radiol 1999;29:503–5.

[46] Tazi K, el Fassi J, Sadiq A, et al. [Major renal trauma: report of 18 cases]. Ann Urol (Paris) 2000; 34:249–53. [French]

[47] Sekiguchi Y, Miyai K, Noguchi K, et al. [Nonoperative management of major blunt renal lacerations with urinary extravasation: report of two cases]. Hinyokika Kiyo 1998;44:875–8. [Japanese]

[48] Rush DS, Nichols RL. Risk of infection following penetrating abdominal trauma: a selective review. Yale J Biol Med 1986;59:395–401.

[49] Meng MV, Mario LA, McAninch JW. Current treatment and outcomes of perinephric abscesses. J Urol 2002;168:1337–40.

[50] Husmann DA, Gilling PJ, Perry MO, et al. Major renal lacerations with a devitalized fragment following blunt abdominal trauma: a comparison between nonoperative (expectant) versus surgical management. J Urol 1993;150:1774–7.

[51] McAninch JW, Carroll PR, Armenakas NA. Renal gunshot wounds: methods of salvage and reconstruction. J Trauma 1993;35:279–83 [discussion: 283–4].

[52] Rosen MA, McAninch JW. Management of combined renal and pancreatic trauma. J Urol 1994; 152:22–5.

[53] Schaeffer AJ. Infections of the urinary tract. In: Walsh PC, editor. Campbell's urology. Philadelphia: Saunders; 2002. p. 515–602.

[54] Armenakas NA, Duckett CP, McAninch JW. Indications for nonoperative management of renal stab wounds. J Urol 1999;161:768–71.

[55] Ersay A, Akgun Y. Experience with renal gunshot injuries in a rural setting. Urology 1999;54:972–5.

[56] Kristjansson A, Pedersen J. Management of blunt renal trauma. Br J Urol 1993;72:692–6.

[57] Safir M, McAninch JW. Management of complex violent trauma to the upper urinary tract. Trauma 1999;1:323–39.

[58] Radwin HM, Fitch WP, Robison JR. A unified concept of renal trauma. J Urol 1976;116:20–2.

[59] Danuser H, Wille S, Zoscher G, et al. How to treat blunt kidney ruptures: primary open surgery or conservative treatment with deferred surgery when necessary? Eur Urol 2001;39:9–14.

[60] Robert M, Drianno N, Muir G, et al. Management of major blunt renal lacerations: surgical or nonoperative approach? Eur Urol 1996;30:335–9.

[61] McAninch JW, Carroll PR. Renal trauma: kidney preservation through improved vascular control—a refined approach. J Trauma 1982;22:285–90.

[62] Narrod JA, Moore EE, Posner M, et al. Nephrectomy following trauma–impact on patient outcome. J Trauma 1985;25:842–4.

[63] Eastham JA, Wilson TG, Ahlering TE. Urological evaluation and management of renal-proximity stab wounds. J Urol 1993;150:1771–3.

[64] Heyns CF, de Klerk DP, de Kock ML. Stab wounds associated with hematuria—a review of 67 cases. J Urol 1983;130:228–31.

[65] Wessells H, Deirmenjian J, McAninch JW. Preservation of renal function after reconstruction for trauma: quantitative assessment with radionuclide scintigraphy. J Urol 1997;157:1583–6.

[66] El-Sherbiny MT, Aboul-Ghar ME, Hafez AT, et al. Late renal functional and morphological

evaluation after non-operative treatment of high-grade renal injuries in children. BJU Int 2004;93: 1053–6.

[67] Keller MS, Eric Coln C, Garza JJ, et al. Functional outcome of nonoperatively managed renal injuries in children. J Trauma 2004;57:108–10 [discussion: 110].

[68] Saidi A, Bocqueraz F, Descotes JL, et al. [Blunt kidney trauma: a ten-year experience]. Prog Urol 2004;14:1125–31. [French]

[69] Bergqvist D, Grenabo L, Hedelin H, et al. Long-time follow-up of patients with conservatively treated blunt renal injuries. Acta Chir Scand 1980; 146:291–4.

[70] Margenthaler JA, Weber TR, Keller MS. Blunt renal trauma in children: experience with conservative management at a pediatric trauma center. J Trauma 2002;52:928–32.

[71] McGonigal MD, Lucas CE, Ledgerwood AM. The effects of treatment of renal trauma on renal function. J Trauma 1987;27:471–6.

[72] Carroll PR, McAninch JW. Operative indications in penetrating renal trauma. J Trauma 1985;25: 587–93.

[73] Barsness KA, Bensard DD, Partrick D, et al. Renovascular injury: an argument for renal preservation. J Trauma 2004;57:310–5.

[74] Watts RA, Hoffbrand BI. Hypertension following renal trauma. J Hum Hypertens 1987;1:65–71.

[75] Nicol AJ, Theunissen D. Renal salvage in penetrating kidney injuries: a prospective analysis. J Trauma 2002;53:351–3.

[76] Grant RP Jr, Gifford RW Jr, Pudvan WR, et al. Renal trauma and hypertension. Am J Cardiol 1971;27:173–6.

[77] Miller KS, McAninch JW. Radiographic assessment of renal trauma: our 15-year experience. J Urol 1995;154:352–5.

[78] Cass AS, Luxenberg M, Gleich P, et al. Long-term results of conservative and surgical management of blunt renal lacerations. Br J Urol 1987;59:17–20.

[79] Mogensen P, Agger P, Ostergaard AH. A conservative approach to the management of blunt renal trauma. Results of a follow-up study. Br J Urol 1980;52:338–41.

[80] Jameson RM. Transient hypertension associated with closed renal injury. Br J Urol 1973;45:482–4.

[81] von Knorring J, Fyhrquist F, Ahonen J. Varying course of hypertension following renal trauma. J Urol 1981;126:798–801.

[82] Meyrier A, Rainfray M, Lacombe M. Delayed hypertension after blunt renal trauma. Am J Nephrol 1988;8:108–11.

[83] Goldblatt H, Lynch J, Hanzal RF, Summerville WW. Studies on experimental hypertension: the production of persistent elevation of systolic blood pressure by means of renal ischemia. J Exp Med 1934;59:347–80.

[84] Montgomery RC, Richardson JD, Harty JI. Post-traumatic renovascular hypertension after occult renal injury. J Trauma 1998;45:106–10.

[85] Monstrey SJ, Beerthuizen GI, vander Werken C, et al. Renal trauma and hypertension. J Trauma 1989;29:65–70.

[86] Lock JS, Carraway RP, Hudson HC Jr, et al. Proper management of renal artery injury from blunt trauma. South Med J 1985;78:406–10.

[87] Stables DP, Fouche RF, de Villiers van Niekerk JP, et al. Traumatic renal artery occlusion: 21 cases. J Urol 1976;115:229–33.

[88] Haas CA, Spirnak JP. Traumatic renal artery occlusion: a review of the literature. Tech Urol 1998;4:1–11.

[89] Detection, evaluation, and treatment of renovascular hypertension. Final report. Working Group on Renovascular Hypertension. Arch Intern Med 1987;147:820–9.

[90] Page IH. Production of perstent arterial hypertension by cellophane perinephritis. JAMA 1939;113: 2046–8.

[91] Engel WJ, Page IH. Hypertension due to renal compression resulting from subcapsular hematoma. J Urol 1955;73:735–9.

[92] Haydar A, Bakri RS, Prime M, et al. Page kidney—a review of the literature. J Nephrol 2003;16:329–33.

[93] McCune TR, Stone WJ, Breyer JA. Page kidney: case report and review of the literature. Am J Kidney Dis 1991;18:593–9.

[94] Aragona F, Artibani W, Calabro A, et al. Page kidney: a curable form of arterial hypertension. Case report and review of the literature. Urol Int 1991; 46:203–7.

[95] Wheatley JK, Motamedi F, Hammonds WD. Page kidney resulting from massive subcapsular hematoma. Complication of lumbar sympathetic nerve block. Urology 1984;24:361–3.

[96] Pintar TJ, Zimmerman S. Hyperreninemic hypertension secondary to a subcapsular perinephric hematoma in a patient with polyarteritis nodosa. Am J Kidney Dis 1998;32:503–7.

[97] Sasaguri M, Noda K, Matsumoto T, et al. A case of hyperreninemic hypertension after extracorporeal shock-wave lithotripsy. Hypertens Res 2000;23: 709–12.

[98] Mufarrij P, Sandhu JS, Coll DM, et al. Page kidney as a complication of percutaneous antegrade endopyelotomy. Urology 2005;65:592.

[99] Matlaga BR, Veys JA, Jung F, et al. Subcapsular urinoma: an unusual form of page kidney in a high school wrestler. J Urol 2002;168:672.

[100] Patel MR, Mooppan MM, Kim H. Subcapsular urinoma: unusual form of "page kidney" in newborn. Urology 1984;23:585–7.

[101] Johnson JD, Radwin HM. High renin hypertension associated with renal cortical cyst. Urology 1976;7: 508–11.

[102] Yussim A, Shmuely D, Levy J, et al. Page kidney phenomenon in kidney allograft following peritransplant lymphocele. Urology 1988;31:512–4.

[103] Kato K, Takashi M, Narita H, et al. Renal hypertension secondary to perirenal pseudocyst: resolution by percutaneous drainage. J Urol 1985;134: 942–3.

[104] Nakano S, Kigoshi T, Uchida K, et al. Hypertension and unilateral renal ischemia (Page kidney) due to compression of a retroperitoneal paraganglioma. Am J Nephrol 1996;16:91–4.

[105] Vasile M, Bellin MF, Helenon O, et al. Imaging evaluation of renal trauma. Abdom Imaging 2000;25:424–30.

[106] Sterns RH, Rabinowitz R, Segal AJ, et al. 'Page kidney'. Hypertension caused by chronic subcapsular hematoma. Arch Intern Med 1985;145: 169–71.

[107] Castle EP, Herrell SD. Laparoscopic management of page kidney. J Urol 2002;168:673–4.

[108] Carroll PR, McAninch JW, Klosterman P. Renovascular trauma: risk assessment, surgical management, and outcome. J Trauma 1990;30:547–52 [discussion: 553].

[109] Cass AS, Bubrick M, Luxenberg M, et al. Renal pedicle injury in patients with multiple injuries. J Trauma 1985;25:892–6.

[110] Turner WW Jr, Snyder WH III, Fry WJ. Mortality and renal salvage after renovascular trauma. A review of 94 patients treated in a 20 year period. Am J Surg 1983;146:848–51.

[111] Knudson MM, Harrison PB, Hoyt DB, et al. Outcome after major renovascular injuries: a Western trauma association multicenter report. J Trauma 2000;49:1116–22.

[112] Bahloul A, Krid M, Trifa M, et al. [Contusions to the pathologic kidney. A retrospective study, apropos of 34 cases]. Ann Urol (Paris) 1997;31: 253–8. [French]

[113] Persky L, Forsythe WE, Forsythe WE III. Trauma and simulated renal disease. J Trauma 1964;128: 197–203.

[114] Cass AS. Blunt renal pelvic and ureteral injury in multiple-injured patients. Urology 1983;22:268–70.

[115] Morse TS, Smith JP, Howard WH, et al. Kidney injuries in children. J Urol 1967;98:539–47.

[116] Presti JC Jr, Carroll PR, McAninch JW. Ureteral and renal pelvic injuries from external trauma: diagnosis and management. J Trauma 1989;29:370–4.

[117] McAleer IM, Kaplan GW, LoSasso BE. Congenital urinary tract anomalies in pediatric renal trauma patients. J Urol 2002;168:1808–10 [discussion: 1810].

[118] Onen A, Kaya M, Cigdem MK, et al. Blunt renal trauma in children with previously undiagnosed pre-existing renal lesions and guidelines for effective initial management of kidney injury. BJU Int 2002;89:936–41.

[119] Wessells H, McAninch JW, Meyer A, et al. Criteria for nonoperative treatment of significant penetrating renal lacerations. J Urol 1997;157:24–7.

[120] Heyns CF, Van Vollenhoven P. Selective surgical management of renal stab wounds. Br J Urol 1992;69:351–7.

[121] Heyns CF, De Klerk DP, De Kock ML. Nonoperative management of renal stab wounds. J Urol 1985;134:239–42.

[122] Teigen CL, Venbrux AC, Quinlan DM, et al. Late massive hematuria as a complication of conservative management of blunt renal trauma in children. J Urol 1992;147:1333–6.

[123] Lee RS, Porter JR. Traumatic renal artery pseudoaneurysm: diagnosis and management techniques. J Trauma 2003;55:972–8.

[124] Chazen MD, Miller KS. Intrarenal pseudoaneurysm presenting 15 years after penetrating renal injury. Urology 1997;49:774–6.

[125] Morin RP, Dunn EJ, Wright CB. Renal arteriovenous fistulas: a review of etiology, diagnosis, and management. Surgery 1986;99:114–8.

[126] Bernath AS, Schutte H, Fernandez RR, et al. Stab wounds of the kidney: conservative management in flank penetration. J Urol 1983;129:468–70.

[127] Ishikawa T, Fujisawa M, Kawabata G, et al. Assessment of availability of magnetic resonance angiography (MRA) in renal arteriovenous fistula. Urol Res 2004;32:104–6.

[128] Darcq C, Guy L, Garcier JM, et al. [Post-traumatic secondary arteriovenous fistulae of the kidney and their embolization. Report of 3 cases.] Prog Urol 2002;12:21–6. [French]

[129] Uflacker R, Paolini RM, Lima S. Management of traumatic hematuria by selective renal artery embolization. J Urol 1984;132:662–7.

[130] Benson DA, Stockinger ZT, McSwain NE Jr. Embolization of an acute renal arteriovenous fistula following a stab wound: case report and review of the literature. Am Surg 2005;71:62–5.

[131] Dinkel HP, Danuser H, Triller J. Blunt renal trauma: minimally invasive management with microcatheter embolization experience in nine patients. Radiology 2002;223:723–30.

[132] Reilly KJ, Shapiro MB, Haskal ZJ. Angiographic embolization of a penetrating traumatic renal arteriovenous fistula. J Trauma 1996;41:763–5.

[133] Tucci P, Doctor D, Diagonale A. Embolization of post-traumatic renal arteriovenous fistula. Urology 1979;13:192–4.

[134] Velmahos GC, Chahwan S, Falabella A, et al. Angiographic embolization for intraperitoneal and retroperitoneal injuries. World J Surg 2000; 24:539–45.

[135] Fisher RG, Ben-Menachem Y, Whigham C. Stab wounds of the renal artery branches: angiographic diagnosis and treatment by embolization. Am J Roentgenol 1989;152:1231–5.

[136] Swana HS, Cohn SM, Burns GA, et al. Renal artery pseudoaneurysm after blunt abdominal trauma: case report and literature review. J Trauma 1996;40:459–61.

[137] Testart J, Watelet J, Poels D. Pseudoaneurysm resulting from avulsion of the right renal artery: endoaneurysmal bypass. Eur J Vasc Surg 1991;5:475–8.

[138] Pinto IT, Chimeno PC. Treatment of a urinoma and a post-traumatic pseudoaneurysm using selective arterial embolization. Cardiovasc Intervent Radiol 1998;21:506–8.

[139] Farrell TM, Sutton JE, Burchard KW. Renal artery pseudoaneurysm: a cause of delayed hematuria in blunt trauma. J Trauma 1996;41:1067–8.

[140] Jebara VA, El Rassi I, Achouh PE, et al. Renal artery pseudoaneurysm after blunt abdominal trauma. J Vasc Surg 1998;27:362–5.

[141] Hassantash SA, Mock C, Maier RV. Traumatic visceral artery aneurysm: presentation as massive hemorrhage from perforation into an adjacent hollow viscus. J Trauma 1995;38:357–60.

[142] Khan AB, Reid AW. Management of renal stab wounds by arteriographic embolisation. Scand J Urol Nephrol 1994;28:109–10.

[143] Chen X, Borsa JJ, Dubinsky T, et al. CT of a renal artery pseudoaneurysm caused by a stab wound. AJR Am J Roentgenol 2002;178:736.

[144] Hemingway AP, Allison DJ. Complications of embolization: analysis of 410 procedures. Radiology 1988;166:669–72.

[145] Beaujeux R, Saussine C, al-Fakir A, et al. Superselective endo-vascular treatment of renal vascular lesions. J Urol 1995;153:14–7.

[146] Chatziioannou A, Brountzos E, Primetis E, et al. Effects of superselective embolization for renal vascular injuries on renal parenchyma and function. Eur J Vasc Endovasc Surg 2004;28:201–6.

[147] DiGiacomo JC, Rotondo MF, Kauder DR, et al. The role of nephrectomy in the acutely injured. Arch Surg 2001;136:1045–9.

[148] Taviloglu K, Gunay K, Ertekin C, et al. Abdominal stab wounds: the role of selective management. Eur J Surg 1998;164:17–21.

[149] Velmahos GC, Demetriades D, Cornwell EE III, et al. Selective management of renal gunshot wounds. Br J Surg 1998;85:1121–4.

[150] Knight CG, Omert L. Chylous ascites after nephrectomy for trauma. Am Surg 2004;70:1083–4.

ELSEVIER
SAUNDERS

Urol Clin N Am 33 (2006) 55–66

UROLOGIC
CLINICS
of North America

Ureteral Injuries: External and Iatrogenic

Sean P. Elliott, MD*, Jack W. McAninch, MD

*Department of Urology, University of California, San Francisco, San Francisco General Hospital,
1001 Potrero Avenue, 3A-20, San Francisco, CA 94110, USA*

Ureteral injuries should be classified as those that present acutely and those that have a more insidious onset. Acute ureteral injury is rare and occurs more commonly intra-operatively (80%) than from external violent trauma (20%). Radiation, ureterolithiasis, and prior instrumentation are a few causes of chronic ureteral injury that presents with fistula or with hydroureteronephrosis secondary to ureteral stricture. This article will concentrate on the etiology, diagnosis, and management of the acute ureteral injury.

Anatomy

The ureter originates from the renal pelvis as the most posterior structure in the renal hilum (Fig. 1). The ureter then travels caudally through the retroperitoneum along the anterior surface of the psoas muscle, posterior to the colonic mesentery and lateral to the gonadal vein. At the pelvic inlet, the gonadal vein crosses the ureter. The ureter then crosses anterior to the common iliac vessels, courses lateral to the internal iliac vessels, and then turns medially, where it is crossed by the vas deferens in the man or the uterine artery in the woman. It finally tunnels in the posterior wall of the bladder.

The blood supply to the ureter comes from the renal artery, gonadal artery, lumbar arteries, and aorta proximally and the internal iliac artery and its branches distally. A delicate network of subadventitial vessels supplies the intervening area.

Types of ureteral injury

Intraoperatively, the ureter can be injured by suture ligation, sharp incision or transection, avulsion, devascularization, and heat (eg, microwave, electrocautery, or vibratory energy) or cryoablative therapy. Injury by transection, ligation, or avulsion may be immediately apparent. Injury in cases of devascularization, heat, or cryoablative therapy may not be apparent because these insults may not immediately result in any change in ureteral patency. For this reason, clinicians must maintain a high degree of suspicion for injury in such cases. In cases involving external violent trauma, the ureter may be injured by blunt avulsion or transection by stab wound or gunshot wound.

Epidemiology and pathogenesis

Iatrogenic ureteral injuries

Gynecologic procedures

According to estimates, 52% to 82% of operative ureteral injuries occur during gynecologic surgery [1–4]. The ureter is more commonly injured during an abdominal hysterectomy (2.2%) [5–7] than a vaginal hysterectomy (0.03%) [8] and more commonly in an open abdominal hysterectomy than in a laparoscopic hysterectomy (1.3%) [9]. This difference may in part be due to a selection bias as hysterectomies complicated by infection and malignancy are approached transabdominally. Risk factors for ureteral injury include a large uterus, pelvic organ prolapse, and prior pelvic surgery [7,10]. The ureter is usually injured as it crosses inferior to the uterine artery. Ureteral injury is not recognized at the time of surgery in 33% to 87.5% of cases [2,7,10,11].

* Corresponding author.
E-mail address: LAYLA@itsa.ucsf.edu (S.P. Elliott).

0094-0143/06/$ - see front matter © 2005 Elsevier Inc. All rights reserved.
doi:10.1016/j.ucl.2005.11.005

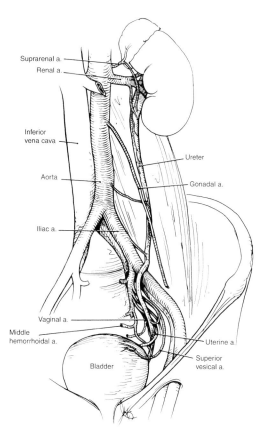

Fig. 1. Anatomy of the retroperitoneum, with attention to the course ureter and its blood supply. (*From* Guerriero WG, Devine CJ. Urologic injuries. Norwalk (CT): Appleton-Century-Crofts; 1984, with permission.)

General surgical procedures

Low anterior resection (LAR) and abdominal perineal resection (APR) of the colon account for 9% of all ureteral injuries [4]. The incidence of ureteral injury during APR or LAR is 0.3% to 5.7% [12]. The left ureter is more commonly injured than the right because it may be elevated with the sigmoid mesentery and mistaken for a mesenteric vessel.

Vascular procedures

Vascular surgery, including aortoiliac and aortofemoral bypass, can result in intraoperative ureteral injury to the mid- and distal third of the ureter. Either surgical devascularization or inflammation can result in delayed recognition of ureteral strictures and catastrophic ureteroiliac fistulas. However, these chronic insults are outside the realm of our discussion.

Urologic procedures

Ureteroscopic ureteral injuries that are acutely recognized range from mucosal false passage or perforation to avulsion and intussusception. Ureteroscopy in the modern era results in ureteral avulsion in 0.3% and perforation in 2% to 6% of cases. Perforation rates are lowest in the most recent series and in those series using smaller caliber ureteroscopes [13–15]. Increased operative time is predictive of injury [13]. Nearly all perforations can be managed with an indwelling ureteral stent without any significant increase in stricture rate compared with the atraumatic ureteroscopic procedure. Open surgical repair of the injured ureter is required after ureteral avulsion or after complicated perforations and occurs in 1.1% of cases [15]. The ureter is at greatest risk for injury from ureteroscopy at the ureterovesical junction, pelvic brim, and the ureteropelvic junction. The muscular backing of the ureter is thin at the ureterovesical junction and ureteropelvic junction. Meanwhile, the angulation of the ureter makes it vulnerable to injury at the pelvic brim.

The ureter is also at risk for injury at the ureteropelvic junction during thermoablation of renal tumors. There may be a higher risk of injury with lower pole and medially located tumors. The ureter may also be at higher risk with microwave therapy than with cryoablation therapy [16,17]. Thermoablation injuries as well as strictures resulting from ureteral balloon dilation, the position of the ureteral access sheath, and renal or ureteral surgery may not be noticed immediately and are outside the realm of this discussion.

Ureteral injuries from external trauma

Because procedures involving the ureter or near the ureter are so frequent, iatrogenic ureteral injury is not uncommon. By comparison, ureteral injuries from external violence are much less common. They represent less than 1% of all genitourinary injuries from violent trauma [18]. Blunt trauma and stab wounds rarely result in injury to the ureter. Blunt trauma represents 4.1% and stab wounds 5.2% of all ureteral traumas. The most common ureteral injuries from external violence are gunshot wounds (90.7%) (Table 1) [18–37]. Still, the ureter is only injured in less than 3% of gunshot wounds to the abdomen [26,33,38]. The relative frequency of ureteral injury from gunshots may be overestimated on an initial literature review because some centers do not report their experience with injuries from stab

Table 1
Mechanism and anatomic location of ureteral trauma: literature reports

Reference	Number of cases	Gunshot wound	Stab wound	Blunt injury	Upper ureter	Mid-ureter	Distal ureter
Elliott [18]	36	22	9	5	25	3	8
Bright [19]	59	52	5	2	19	23	17
Brandes [20]	12	8	4	NPS	2	7	3
Campbell [21]	15	12	0	3	7	4	4
Carlton [22]	39	36	1	2	NA	NA	NA
DiGiacomo [23]	23	23	NPS	NPS	NA	NA	NA
Eikenberg [24]	17	17	NPS	NPS	6	2	9
Ghali [25]	8	2	0	6	7	0	1
Holden [26]	63	63	NPS	NPS	20	27	16
Lankford [27]	10	10	NPS	NPS	6	3	1
Liroff [28]	20	20	NPS	NPS	5	11	4
Medina [29]	20	15	4	1	NA	NA	NA
Palmer [30]	20	19	1	NPS	3	7	10
Perez-Brayfield [31]	55	55	NPS	NPS	23	11	21
Peterson [32]	18	17	1	NPS	5	7	6
Azimuddin [33]	21	19	2	NPS	6	8	7
Stutzman [34]	22	22	NPS	NPS	6	3	13
Steers [35]	18	17	0	1	12	4	2
Rober [36]	16	16	NPS	NPS	8	4	4
Velmahos [37]	41	39	2	NPS	NA	NA	NA
Walker [38]	27	24	0	3	10	12	5
Totals	560	508 (90.7%)	29 (5.2%)	23 (4.1%)	170 (39%)	136 (31%)	131 (30%)

Abbreviations: NPS, not part of study; NA, not available.

wounds and blunt trauma. When taking into consideration only those series that report all three mechanisms of injury, then gunshot wounds account for 81%, stab wounds 9%, and blunt injuries 10% of cases involving ureteral injuries from external violence. Thus, gunshot wounds still represent the predominant mechanism for injuries of this nature.

An understanding of the characteristics of each type of injury is important because etiology, in part, dictates management. Blunt ureteral injury presents after a fall from a height or secondary to a high-speed motor-vehicle accident. Rapid deceleration results in disruption of the ureter at fixed points along its course. Those points are the ureterovesical junction or, more commonly, the ureteropelvic junction, and damage is minimal to the surrounding ureteral segments. Injury to the ureter from stab wounds must be considered in all cases involving stab wounds to the back or stab wounds to the abdomen with a long blade. Again, the injury is usually to a short segment of ureter. Gunshot wounds differ not only in the acuity of the patient at presentation but also in the length of the affected ureter. The cavitation injury from high-velocity projectiles creates a blast effect resulting in thrombosis of the surrounding ureter,

which, on first evaluation, may appear entirely normal. This effect was shown experimentally by Amato et al, who studied gross and microscopic changes after ballistic injury to an isolated segment of ureter in a military laboratory. As much as 2 cm of microscopic vascular damage was documented beyond the limits of gross ureteral injury from a gunshot [39].

Presentation and evaluation

Iatrogenic ureteral injuries

Many ureteral injuries go unrecognized at the time of injury. In fact, of all recognized iatrogenic ureteral injuries, 50% to 70% are not recognized acutely [2,11]. Minor injuries may heal without sequelae. However, when not repaired, significant injuries result in fever, flank pain, nausea, and vomiting from hydronephrosis, urinoma, or ureteral fistula. To avoid a delay in diagnosis, every effort should be made to fully evaluate the ureters intraoperatively in cases at risk for ureteral injury.

Intraoperative evaluation for iatrogenic ureteral injury must be tailored for the clinical situation. The approach depends on the hemodynamic stability of the patient, the positioning of the patient on the operating table, and the surgical approach (eg, endoscopic, laparoscopic, transabdominal, or transvaginal) that resulted in the suspected ureteral injury. When the abdomen is open, the clinician can mobilize and inspect the ureters in the area of suspected injury. Another technique is intravenous or direct renal pelvis injection of methylene blue followed by either direct inspection of the mobilized ureters for leakage or cystoscopic visualization of dye exiting from the ureteral orifices. Ureteral catheters can be passed up the ureters either cystoscopically or through a cystotomy. Easy passage means that ureteral injury is unlikely. Cystoscopy with retrograde pyelograms is sensitive and allows stenting of minor injuries. However, practical limitations to retrograde pyelography include supine positioning of the patients, which can make cystoscopy difficult, and the position of the operating table, which may make placement of a fluoroscopy C-arm impossible. What follows is a limited description of certain clinical situations and a suggested approach for each.

Total vaginal hysterectomy

Total vaginal hysterectomy is done in the lithotomy position, making cystoscopy with ureteral catheterization or observation for excretion of intravenous dye the preferred methods for finding ureteral injuries. Table positioning usually prevents fluoroscopic examination. There have been mixed results using routine cystoscopy with methylene blue intravenous injection after hysterectomy for the detection of ureteral injury [7,10]. Given the low incidence of ureteral injury and the low sensitivity for detecting injury with this method, it is not recommended as standard practice after every procedure. These methods should be reserved for cases in which one suspects an injury. If one suspects an injury based on the results of these tests, then the ureters should be explored through an abdominal incision and repaired.

Total abdominal hysterectomy

When a ureteral injury is suspected during a total abdominal hysterectomy, the ureters should be explored and visually inspected. Intravenous or direct renal pelvis injection of methylene blue may be helpful.

Cesarean section

Ureteral injury can occur during lateral extension of the uterine myotomy into the broad ligament to facilitate fetal delivery. In 69% of cases of intraoperative urologic consultation in one series, the cesarean section was done on an emergency basis [40]. Associated bleeding and the size of the gravid uterus can make visual inspection of the ureters difficult and ureteral mobilization hazardous. In addition, the hydronephrosis associated with the third trimester can make visual inspection for peristalsis or excretion of methylene blue poor indicators of injury. Because of these difficulties and the low incidence of ureteral injuries compared with the number of urologic consultations requested (1 out of 17 in one series [40]), the authors favor ureteral catheterization either cystoscopically or through a cystotomy for the diagnosis of ureteral injuries during cesarean section. The catheters can be left for 1 to 3 days postoperatively and the outputs followed. If one still suspects an injury based on low-volume or bloody catheter output, then a retrograde pyelogram can be done postoperatively.

Laparoscopy

In experienced hands, the ureters can be explored and repaired with laparoscopic techniques. However, one should have a low threshold for making an abdominal incision and performing open ureteral identification and repair [41,42]. In cases necessitating an open incision for organ extraction, it may be possible to design the extraction incision to allow open repair of the ureter as well.

Ureteroscopy

Most ureteroscopic ureteral injuries can be managed with insertion of an indwelling ureteral stent. However, in the case of avulsion, the injury should be immediately repaired transabdominally.

Ureteral injuries from external trauma

The ureters are well protected in the retroperitoneum and great violence must be inflicted to injure the ureter. Therefore, the patient with a ureteral injury is often acutely ill. Hypotension is present in 56% of cases and major organ injury accompanies ureteral injury in greater than 90% of cases [18]. Concomitant injuries most often involve the small and large bowel. However, thoracic and major vascular injuries are common as well [18,22,24,28,32,33,35,43]. While hypotension is common, it is not uniformly present and is indicative of associated injuries rather than the ureteral injury itself.

Hematuria

Either gross or microscopic (ie, >5 red blood cells per high-power field) hematuria is present in 74% of cases of ureteral injury. Gross hematuria is reported in 46% of patients and only microscopic hematuria in 38% [18–36,38,43]. Reasons for the absence of hematuria may include an adynamic partially transected ureter or a complete ureteral transection. While hematuria is frequently present, its absence does not rule out an injury.

Location of injury

Traumatic ureteral injuries occur in the upper ureter in 39% of cases, mid-ureter in 31%, and distal ureter in 30% (Table 1) [18–36,38,43]. A possible reason for the slight predominance of upper ureteral injuries may be that the distal ureter is better protected by the bony pelvis. In addition, the assailant may preferentially aim his or her weapon in the abdomen rather than the pelvis in an effort to hit other vital organs. Most injuries involve a short-segment loss of ureter. An understanding of the location and length of injury is important as this determines the type of reconstruction. Distal ureteral injuries are best repaired with ureteroneocystostomy. While mid- and upper ureteral injuries may occasionally benefit from transureteroureterostomy or a Boari flap procedure, such complex reconstructions are rarely needed and may be inappropriate in the unstable trauma patient. The length of ureteral loss is usually short and the injury can be repaired with mobilization and ureteroureterostomy [18].

Imaging

The most sensitive radiographic study for the diagnosis of ureteral injury is a retrograde pyelogram. However, such a time-consuming study is inappropriate in most trauma situations. Likewise, an intravenous pyelogram (IVP) performed formally in the radiology suite may be a sensitive indicator of injury, but it too costs valuable time in the critically ill trauma patient. Therefore, more appropriate studies include an abbreviated IVP or CT with delayed imaging and pyelography (CT-IVP). Findings suggestive of ureteral injury include extravasation of contrast, hydronephrosis, or nonvisualization of the ureter.

An abdominal CT scan is the gold standard for diagnosis of abdominal injuries after blunt trauma. Therefore, after blunt trauma where ureter injury is suspected, the prudent choice is a CT-IVP because delayed imaging with pyelography can easily be incorporated into the CT scan with only 10 to 15 minutes of extra time. In limited experience, CT-IVPs have proved to be a highly sensitive indicators of ureteral injury after blunt trauma. CT-IVPs correctly identified blunt ureteral injuries in four out of four patients in one series [18]. A CT-IVP is already indicated for the staging of renal trauma in the blunt injury patient with gross hematuria or microscopic hematuria with hypotension [44]. Imaging the blunt trauma patient who meets these criteria will likewise identify the rare ureteral injury.

Victims of penetrating injuries to the abdomen frequently progress immediately to laparotomy for assessment and management of nonurologic intra-abdominal injuries. A CT-IVP and a retrograde pyelogram are impractical in this situation. However, a "one-shot IVP" may be performed without delaying surgical intervention. The one-shot IVP allows the urologist to stage upper urinary tract injuries and confirm bilateral functioning renal moieties. The one-shot IVP involves a single abdominal film taken on the trauma gurney or the operating table 10 minutes after the injection of a 2 cc/kg bolus of intravenous contrast up to a maximum dosage of 150 cc [45]. In the stable penetrating trauma patient who is to be managed nonoperatively, the decision as to which imaging study to perform should be made in concert with imaging and operative plans for other abdominal injuries. If either microscopic hematuria with hypotension or gross hematuria is present, then a CT-IVP is the indicated study for concomitant evaluation of renal trauma.

The experience in the literature with imaging of ureteral injuries is mostly confined to IVP, with CT-IVP and retrograde pyelogram being done in only a few instances in each study. This emphasis on IVPs reflects the fact that gunshots cause the overwhelming majority of ureteral trauma and such patients progress immediately to laparotomy. Overall, IVP predicts injury accurately in 61% of cases. However, such a statistic does not convey the disparity of results at different institutions [18–36,38,43]. Sensitivity ranges from 0% to 100%. This disparity most likely reflects differences in technique when performing an abbreviated IVP in the trauma bay or the operating room. Most studies do not describe the technique used in obtaining an IVP. The single-shot IVP has become the standard for diagnosis of upper urinary tract injuries at San Francisco General Hospital. The single-shot IVP is useful for the diagnosis of renal injury as it can obviate renal exploration in 32% of patients [45]. However, sensitivity for detecting ureteral injury was only 38% with this technique [18]. While a positive IVP can be helpful, a negative study should not prevent one from surgically exploring the ureter when an injury is suspected.

Intraoperative evaluation

Retroperitoneal surgical exploration with direct visual inspection remains the best indicator of ureteral injury. Use of preoperative IVP or CT-IVP varies from institution to institution, as does the quality of related studies. Still, intraoperative inspection, rather than pyelography, detects an average of 89.3% (range 33%–100%) of ureteral injuries [23]. When the path of the missile is in proximity to the ureter, the ureter should be mobilized along its course and examined. One should inspect the wall of the ureter for continuity, hemorrhage, and contusion. Neither blind palpation nor the observation of ureteral peristalsis is a reliable indicator of a healthy ureter. Indigo carmine or methylene blue can be given intravenously and the ureters inspected for leakage of dye. However, in the hypotensive trauma patient, it is often more expeditious to inject the dye directly into the renal pelvis or in a retrograde fashion if the bladder is open. Missed injuries are associated with an increased incidence of complications [18]. Therefore, a thorough assessment is imperative.

Management

After staging the traumatic or iatrogenic ureteral injury, the plan for repair should be based on the length and location of the injury, the patient's overall status, and the associated injuries. While an excellent reconstruction might be possible, a more conservative approach, such as ureteral ligation or stenting, might be more appropriate in the unstable patient. Most injuries are short and can be repaired with debridement and either ureteroneocystostomy in the distal ureter or ureteroureterostomy in the mid- and proximal ureter. Partial transections of the ureteral wall can be managed with primary closure with good results [18]. However, any degree of injury after a gunshot wound or thermal injury requires wide debridement as the degree of microvascular damage can extend for 2 cm beyond evidence of gross injury [39].

The principles of ureteral repair are as follows: (1) Mobilization of the ureter with care to preserve the adventitia, (2) debridement of nonviable tissue to a bleeding edge, and (3) a spatulated, tension-free anastomosis over an internal stent. The authors use interrupted 5-0 absorbable sutures and believe optical magnification to be important to ensure urothelium-to-urothelium apposition. Omental interposition can be used to separate the repair from associated intra-abdominal injuries or intestinal-vaginal suture lines. The surrounding retroperitoneum should be drained.

Distal ureteral injuries

Ureteroneocystostomy

Approximately one third of traumatic injuries and the majority of operative injuries occur in the distal ureter. These injuries are frequently associated with injuries to or ligature of the internal iliac artery or its branches, thus jeopardizing the blood supply to the distal ureter. Therefore, distal ureteral injuries are best repaired by ureteroneocystostomy. The distal ureter, which remains attached to the native ureteral orifice, need not be resected, nor does it need to be ligated unless there is reason to suspect vesicoureteral reflux. The free end of the proximal ureter is debrided, spatulated, and tunneled in the bladder wall in the fashion of Politano-Leadbetter. The origin of the tunnel should be superior and medial to the native ureteral orifice. Placement in the more mobile lateral bladder wall is discouraged as this may result in ureteral kinking. The tunnel should be developed in the direction of the bladder neck and the length of the tunnel should be three times the diameter of the ureter (Fig. 2). Older or hemodynamically unstable patients may benefit from a more rapidly performed refluxing anastomosis. The authors place a double-J ureteral stent, suprapubic tube, and Foley catheter. The Foley catheter can be removed when the urine is clear. The suprapubic tube can be removed in 7 to 10 days and the stent should remain for 6 to 8 weeks.

Vesico-psoas hitch

More extensive loss of distal ureteral length can be bridged with a vesico-psoas hitch. The bladder is mobilized in the space of Retzius. Ligating the contralateral superior vesical pedicle aids in mobilization. The bladder is opened vertically and tented up against the ipsilateral psoas muscle by placing two fingers in the bladder. Nonabsorbable monofilament sutures are placed in the bladder wall outside the epithelium and in the psoas muscle away from the genitofemoral nerve (Fig. 3). The ureter is reimplanted into the bladder as described above.

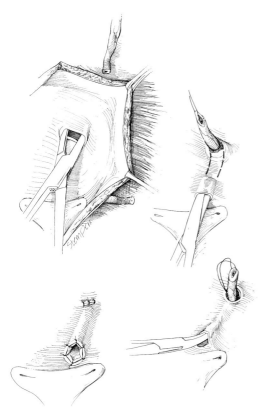

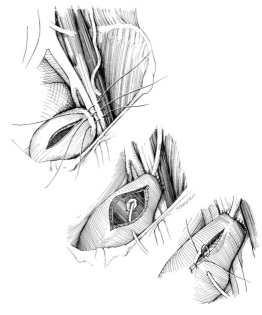

Fig. 3. Ureteroneocystostomy with vesico-psoas hitch. (*From* Presti JC Jr, Carroll PR. Interoperative management of the injured ureter. In: Schrock TR, editor. Perspectives in colon and rectal surgery. St. Louis (MO): Quality Medical Publishing; 1988, with permission from Thieme Medical Publishers, New York.)

Fig. 2. Ureteroneocystostomy in a fashion modified from Politano and Leadbetter. (*From* Presti JC Jr, Carroll PR. Interoperative management of the injured ureter. In: Schrock TR, editor. Perspectives in colon and rectal surgery. St. Louis (MO): Quality Medical Publishing; 1988, with permission from Thieme Medical Publishers, New York.)

Upper and mid-ureteral injuries

Ureteroureterostomy

Frequently, the ureteral segment injured is short. This means that after ureteral debridement and mobilization along the ureter's course, the mid- and proximal ureter can usually be repaired primarily (Fig. 4). In fact, this repair is the most commonly performed type of repair for upper and mid-ureteral injuries [18–21,23–25,26,28–32, 34–36,43]. Before spatulation, a holding suture can be placed on both of the free ends to minimize handling of the ureter with forceps. Likewise, the holding sutures can be used to hold the two ends of ureter together during anastomosis to take some additional tension off the repair. In the past, the anastomosis was performed with running suture to ensure a watertight seal; a nephrostomy

[19] or proximal ureterotomy and externalized T-tube [24] decompressed the ureter in the area of the repair. Today, an interrupted anastomosis is performed over an internalized stent with good results. Ensure that the ends of the ureteral stent are placed in the renal pelvis and bladder as intended. The stent can be palpated in the renal pelvis without difficulty. However, placement in the bladder is often difficult to confirm by palpation. Another way to confirm placement is to fill the bladder with methylene blue through the urethral catheter and observe reflux of blue urine up the stent. Alternatively, cystoscopy can be done to confirm stent position. A plain abdominal radiograph showing the kidneys, ureter, and bladder should be performed postoperatively to confirm stent positioning.

Primary closure

Partial ureteral transections can be closed primarily with good results. The edges of the ureteral wound are debrided and an interrupted closure is performed, preferably over a stent. This type of repair is inappropriate after a gunshot

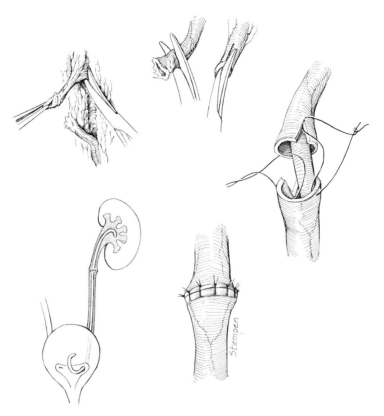

Fig. 4. Ureteroureterostomy demonstrating the principles of debridement, spatulation and end-to-end repair using interrupted, absorbable, fine sutures over an indwelling stent. (*From* Presti JC Jr, Carroll PR. Interoperative management of the injured ureter. In: Schrock TR, editor. Perspectives in colon and rectal surgery. St. Louis (MO): Quality Medical Publishing; 1988, with permission from Thieme Medical Publishers, New York.)

wound or iatrogenic thermal injury because more extensive debridement is necessary.

Transureteroureterostomy

Due to the typically short length of ureteral loss, transureteroureterostomy is rarely indicated. The length of tissue loss can usually be bridged with the simpler maneuvers mentioned above. Occasionally, the ureter may be mistaken intraoperatively for a vessel and a significant length may be resected. In the authors' experience, this error occurs more commonly on the left side where the ureter is mistaken for the ascending inferior mesenteric vein. Likewise, in the trauma setting, after more extensive ureteral loss or when pelvic injuries preclude ureteroneocystostomy (eg, rectal injury, major vascular injury, or extensive bladder injury), transureteroureterostomy is an excellent option. The donor ureter should be generously mobilized. However, care must be

taken not to compromise the longitudinal vessels running in the adventitial layer. The recipient ureter should be mobilized as little as possible to ensure adequate blood supply to the anastomosis. The donor ureter should be tunneled through the sigmoid colon mesentery superior to the inferior mesenteric artery to avoid kinking. A small ellipse is excised from the medial wall of the recipient ureter. The donor ureter is spatulated and an end-to-side anastomosis is performed (Fig. 5). A double-J stent should be placed from the donor kidney, across the anastomosis, and down to the bladder. If the recipient ureter is wide enough, a second stent can be placed from the recipient kidney to the bladder. However, the placing of a second stent is not imperative. The only absolute contraindications to transureteroureterostomy include inadequate ureteral length and a diseased recipient ureter. Relative contraindications include a history of nephrolithiasis or pelvic

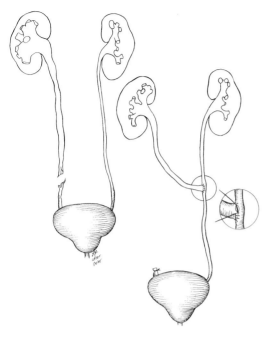

Fig. 5. Transureteroureterostomy. (*From* Presti JC Jr, Carroll PR. Ureteral and renal pelvic trauma: diagnosis and management. In: McAninch JW, editor. Traumatic and reconstructive urology. Philadelphia: W.B. Saunders; 1996. p. 178, with permission.)

radiation. If the renal unit on the side of the injured ureter is known to have minimal function, then a transureteroureterostomy is discouraged because the procedure may compromise drainage of the dominant kidney. In such a case, nephrectomy may be preferable.

Boari tubularized bladder flap

The Boari tubularized bladder flap is an excellent means of bridging long gaps in ureteral continuity (Fig. 6). However, the procedure for using this flap is time-consuming and best reserved for the stable patient or the elective reconstruction setting. Usually, the loss of ureteral length is short enough that complex repairs such as the Boari flap are not necessary. The authors have performed one Boari flap reconstruction in the acute trauma setting for a man with two ipsilateral complete ureteral transactions. In this rare setting, the intervening ureter is at risk of being nonviable and should be resected, resulting in a long defect, which in this case was best repaired with a Boari flap.

Autotransplantation and ileal ureter

Procedures involving autotransplantation and an ileal ureter are not appropriate in the acute trauma setting and are rarely indicated at the time of intraoperative consultation for ureteral injury. Ureteral defects so extensive as to make one consider autotransplantation or an ileal ureter should be temporized with ureteral ligation and a nephrostomy tube, allowing the case at hand to be completed and the urologist to have a discussion with the patient about options for elective repair. The authors do not place the nephrostomy tube in the operating room because its use too can be time-consuming. Rather, the authors prefer that it be placed on a semi-elective basis in the next 2 to 3 days.

Complications

The incidence of complications after the repair of the iatrogenically injured ureter is not reported. However, the complication rate after repair of traumatic injuries of the ureter is 25% [18–20, 22–36,38,43]. Prolonged urinary leakage at the anastomosis is the most common acute genitourinary complication. Presentation can include urinoma, abscess, or peritonitis. Placement of a drain in the retroperitoneum at the time of initial repair is a preventive measure because it allows efflux of urine in case of leakage and it helps clinicians recognize the leakage earlier. High-volume output from the drain should be measured for creatinine level. Delayed recognition of undrained leakage at the anastomosis is associated with additional morbidity, such as sepsis, more complicated reconstruction, and prolonged hospital stay [18,21,26,29,38]. Delayed urologic complications include ureteral stricture and retained ureteral stent leading to stone formation [18]. Follow-up can be particularly difficult in the trauma setting due to the transient nature of the patient population. Therefore, a true assessment of the incidence of long-term complications is difficult. Acute nonurologic complications and death from other causes are also common in patients with traumatic ureteral injury because of the gravity of associated injuries and not because of the ureteral injury itself. As is well documented in trauma literature, delayed recognition of any traumatic injury leads to an increased complication rate [46]. Likewise, delayed recognition of ureteral injury has led to undrained urinoma, urosepsis, and a more complicated repair [18].

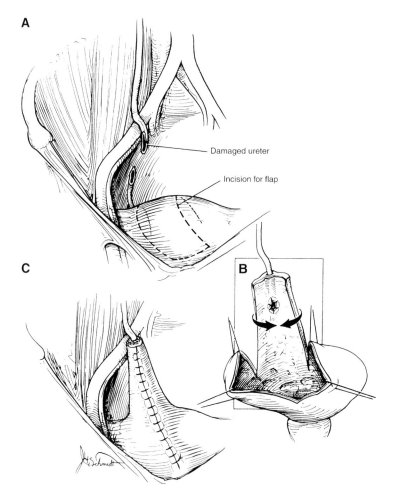

Fig. 6. (*A–C*) Boari tubularized bladder flap and ureteroneocystostomy. (*From* Guerriero WG, Devine CJ. Urologic injuries. Norwalk (CT): Appleton-Century-Crofts; 1984, with permission.)

Summary

Both iatrogenic and traumatic ureteral injuries are rare. Missed ureteral injuries are associated with increased morbidity. Therefore a high index of suspicion is warranted. The urologist should be familiar with several methods of identifying ureteral injuries and the evaluation should be tailored to the clinical situation. Most ureteral injuries are short transections and can be repaired with debridement and ureteroureterostomy in the proximal and mid-ureter or with ureteroneocystostomy in the distal ureter.

References

[1] Lee RA, Symmonds RE, Williams TJ. Current status of genitourinary fistula. Obstet Gynecol 1988; 72(3 Pt 1):313–9.

[2] Dowling RA, Corriere JN Jr, Sandler CM. Iatrogenic ureteral injury. J Urol 1986;135(5):912–5.

[3] Rock J, Thompson JD. Operative injuries to the ureter: prevention, recognition and managment. In: Te Linde's operative gynecology. 8th edition. Philadelphia: Lippincott-Raven; 1997. p. 1137–9.

[4] St Lezin MA, Stoller ML. Surgical ureteral injuries. Urology 1991;38(6):497–506.

[5] Riss P, Koelbl H, Neunteufel W, et al. Wertheim radical hysterectomy 1921–1986: changes in urologic complications. Arch Gynecol Obstet 1988;241(4): 249–53.

[6] Larson DM, Malone JM Jr, Copeland LJ, et al. Ureteral assessment after radical hysterectomy. Obstet Gynecol 1987;69(4):612–6.

[7] Vakili B, Chesson RR, Kyle BL, et al. The incidence of urinary tract injury during hysterectomy: a prospective analysis based on universal cystoscopy. Am J Obstet Gynecol 2005;192(5):1599–604.

[8] Mathevet P, Valencia P, Cousin C, et al. Operative injuries during vaginal hysterectomy. Eur J Obstet Gynecol Reprod Biol 2001;97(1):71–5.

[9] Harkki-Siren P, Sjoberg J, Tiitinen A. Urinary tract injuries after hysterectomy. Obstet Gynecol 1998; 92(1):113–8.

[10] Dandolu V, Mathai E, Chatwani A, et al. Accuracy of cystoscopy in the diagnosis of ureteral injury in benign gynecologic surgery. Int Urogynecol J Pelvic Floor Dysfunct 2003;14(6):427–31.

[11] Ostrzenski A, Radolinski B, Ostrzenska KM. A review of laparoscopic ureteral injury in pelvic surgery. Obstet Gynecol Surv 2003;58(12):794–9.

[12] Coburn M. Ureteral injuries from surgical trauma. In: McAninch JW, editor. Traumatic and reconstructive urology. Philadelphia: W.B. Saunders; 1996. p. 181–97.

[13] Schuster TG, Hollenbeck BK, Faerber GJ, et al. Complications of ureteroscopy: analysis of predictive factors. J Urol 2001;166(2):538–40.

[14] Johnson DB, Pearle MS. Complications of ureteroscopy. Urol Clin North Am 2004;31(1): 157–71.

[15] Stoller ML, Wolf JS Jr. Endoscopic ureteral injuries. In: McAninch JW, editor. Traumatic and reconstructive urology. Philadelphia: W.B. Saunders; 1996. p. 199–211.

[16] Harabayashi T, Shinohara N, Kakizaki H, et al. Ureteral stricture developing after partial nephrectomy with a microwave tissue coagulator: case report. J Endourol 2003;17(10):919–21.

[17] Brashears JH 3rd, Raj GV, Crisci A, et al. Renal cryoablation and radio frequency ablation: an evaluation of worst case scenarios in a porcine model. J Urol 2005;173(6):2160–5.

[18] Elliott SP, McAninch JW. Ureteral injuries from external violence: the 25-year experience at San Francisco General Hospital. J Urol 2003;170(4 Pt 1): 1213–6.

[19] Bright TC 3rd, Peters PC. Ureteral injuries due to external violence: 10 years' experience with 59 cases. J Trauma 1977;17(8):616–20.

[20] Brandes SB, Chelsky MJ, Buckman RF, et al. Ureteral injuries from penetrating trauma. J Trauma 1994;36(6):766–9.

[21] Campbell EW Jr, Filderman PS, Jacobs SC. Ureteral injury due to blunt and penetrating trauma. Urology 1992;40(3):216–20.

[22] Carlton CE Jr, Scott R Jr, Guthrie AG. The initial management of ureteral injuries: a report of 78 cases. J Urol 1971;105(3):335–40.

[23] Digiacomo JC, Frankel H, Rotondo MF, et al. Preoperative radiographic staging for ureteral injuries is not warranted in patients undergoing celiotomy for trauma. Am Surg 2001;67(10): 969–73.

[24] Eickenberg H, Amin M. Gunshot wounds to the ureter. J Trauma 1976;16(7):562–5.

[25] Ghali AM, El Malik EM, Ibrahim AI, et al. Ureteric injuries: diagnosis, management, and outcome. J Trauma 1999;46(1):150–8.

[26] Holden S, Hicks CC, O'Brien DP, et al. Gunshot wounds of the ureter: a 15-year review of 63 consecutive cases. J Urol 1976;116(5):562–4.

[27] Lankford R, Block NL, Politano VA. Gunshot wounds of the ureter: a review of 10 cases. J Trauma 1974;14(10):848–52.

[28] Liroff SA, Pontes JE, Pierce JM Jr. Gunshot wounds of the ureter: 5 years of experience. J Urol 1977; 118(4):551–3.

[29] Medina D, Lavery R, Ross SE, et al. Ureteral trauma: preoperative studies neither predict injury nor prevent missed injuries. J Am Coll Surg 1998; 186(6):641–4.

[30] Palmer LS, Rosenbaum RR, Gershbaum MD, et al. Penetrating ureteral trauma at an urban trauma center: 10-year experience. Urology 1999;54(1): 34–6.

[31] Perez-Brayfield MR, Keane TE, Krishnan A, et al. Gunshot wounds to the ureter: a 40-year experience at Grady Memorial Hospital. J Urol 2001;166(1): 119–21.

[32] Peterson NE, Pitts JC 3rd. Penetrating injuries of the ureter. J Urol 1981;126(5):587–90.

[33] Azimuddin K, Milanesa D, Ivatury R, et al. Penetrating ureteric injuries. Injury 1998;29(5):363–7.

[34] Stutzman RE. Ballistics and the management of ureteral injuries from high velocity missiles. J Urol 1977; 118(6):947–9.

[35] Steers WD, Corriere JN Jr, Benson GS, et al. The use of indwelling ureteral stents in managing ureteral injuries due to external violence. J Trauma 1985; 25(10):1001–3.

[36] Rober PE, Smith JB, Pierce JM Jr. Gunshot injuries of the ureter. J Trauma 1990;30(1):83–6.

[37] Velmahos GC, Degiannis E. The management of urinary tract injuries after gunshot wounds of the anterior and posterior abdomen. Injury 1997;28(8): 535–8.

[38] Walker JA. Injuries of the ureter due to external violence. J Urol 1969;102(4):410–3.

[39] Amato JJ, Billy LJ, Gruber RP, et al. Vascular injuries. An experimental study of high and low velocity missile wounds. Arch Surg 1970;101(2):167–74.

[40] Yossepowitch O, Baniel J, Livne PM. Urological injuries during cesarean section: intraoperative diagnosis and management. J Urol 2004;172(1): 196–9.

[41] Branco AW, Branco Filho AJ, Kondo W. Laparocopic ureteral reimplantation in ureteral stenosis after gynecologic laparoscopic surgery. Int Braz J Urol 2005;31(1):51–3.

[42] Ou CS, Huang IA, Rowbotham R. Laparoscopic ureteroureteral anastomosis for repair of ureteral injury involving stricture. Int Urogynecol J Pelvic Floor Dysfunct 2005;16(2):155–7 [discussion: 157].

[43] Velmahos GC, Degiannis E, Wells M, et al. Penetrating ureteral injuries: the impact of associated injuries on management. Am Surg 1996;62(6):461-8.

[44] McAninch J, Santucci RA, et al. Genitourinary trauma. In: Walsh PC, Retik AB, Vaughan ED Jr, editors. Campbell's urology. 8th edition. Philadelphia: W.B. Saunders; 2002.

[45] Morey AF, McAninch JW, Tiller BK, et al. Single shot intraoperative excretory urography for the immediate evaluation of renal trauma. J Urol 1999; 161(4):1088-92.

[46] Scalea TM, Phillips TF, Goldstein AS, et al. Injuries missed at operation: nemesis of the trauma surgeon. J Trauma 1988;28(7):962-7.

ELSEVIER
SAUNDERS

Urol Clin N Am 33 (2006) 67–71

UROLOGIC
CLINICS
of North America

Diagnosis and Management of Bladder Injuries

Joseph N. Corriere Jr., MD[a,b,*], Carl M. Sandler, MD[a,b]

[a]The University of Texas MD Anderson Cancer Center, Houston, TX, USA
[b]The University of Texas Medical School, Houston, TX, USA

In 2002, a consensus statement on bladder injuries was constructed by an international panel that met in conjunction with the biannual meeting of the Societe Internationale D'Urologie in Stockholm, Sweden. The report was later published in the *British Journal of Urology International* in 2004 and is well accepted as the proper way to diagnose and treat injuries to the urinary bladder [1].

Anatomy and mechanism of injury

In the adult, when the bladder is empty, the bony pelvis protects it from blunt injury, but when full it rises into the lower abdomen and is vulnerable to rupture at the dome by a direct blow. The bladder in the child is almost entirely an abdominal organ and more easily ruptured at less than capacity.

If the pelvis is fractured a spicule of bone may puncture the bladder or, more likely, the shearing force of the attachments of the bladder to bone may tear it during disruption of the pelvic ring.

Although stated in many reports that most injuries associated with pelvic fractures occur adjacent to the fracture, this is seen only 35% of the time. In the other 65% of cases, no relationship exists between the fracture and site of the bladder injury and the injury is commonly opposite the area of the fracture, implying that a bursting injury or tearing of the bladder wall is the true mechanism rather than laceration by

bone [2–4]. Missles of any type can injure the bladder despite its level of distention.

Etiology

Most blunt bladder injuries are caused by a blow to the abdomen secondary to motor vehicle accidents, falls, or a heavy object falling on an individual. In motor vehicle accidents, the unrestrained occupant may be thrown against an unyielding object or the passenger wearing a seat belt may have the force of the collision focus on the lower abdomen during deceleration, especially when the bladder is full [4,5].

Penetrating injuries caused by external violence are caused most commonly by gunshot wounds but may also be caused by knives or spike impalement. Overall, the most common lesions are iatrogenic but may also occur from erosion of internally placed foreign material or swallowed objects. Below is a list of penetrating injury etiologies [4].

Operative injury
  Transurethral procedures
  Gynecologic procedures
  Abdominal procedures
  Orthopedic procedures
Internal erosion
  Surgical drains
  Sterilization devices
  Hip prostheses
  Penile prostheses
  Neurosurgic shunts
  Foley catheters
Swallowed objects
External violence
  Gunshot
  Knife
  Spike impalement

* Corresponding author. 1220 Holcombe Boulevard, Unit 1274, Houston, TX 77030.
  E-mail address: jcorriere@mail.mdanderson.org (J.N. Corriere, Jr).

0094-0143/06/$ - see front matter © 2005 Elsevier Inc. All rights reserved.
doi:10.1016/j.ucl.2005.10.003

urologic.theclinics.com

Signs and symptoms

Gross hematuria is the hallmark of a bladder injury occurring over 95% of the time [6,7]. In the other cases, microscopic hematuria is present. Usually the patient has nonspecific complaints, such as suprapubic pain or if he or she attempts to urinate cannot. Tenderness may be present over the pelvis if it is fractured. In women, if the vagina is injured also, blood and occasionally urine may come from the vagina. Adequate speculum examination is mandatory in these cases and radiographic documentation should be done before suturing of any vaginal lacerations. If diagnosis is delayed, an ileus, uroacities and signs of peritonitis may develop.

Radiographic examination

A retrograde static cystogram performed by filling the bladder with contrast through a urethral catheter is the only definitive study to diagnose a ruptured bladder. In men, if a urethral injury is suspected, a retrograde urethrogram should be considered before placing a urethral catheter [8]. Imaging of the bladder using only excreted contrast material by CT or by conventional radiography is not adequate and results in false-negative studies [9–11]. On a conventional cystogram, the area behind the bladder should be imaged after the instilled contrast has been drained to obviate missing extravasation obscured by the intravesical contrast [12]. When a CT cystogram is performed, this is unnecessary.

If a urethral rupture is found and a suprapubic tube is placed as initial therapy, the bladder still must be examined for a concomitant injury. If the tube is placed percutaneously, a static cystogram then should be performed as described above. If placed surgically, the entire bladder should be inspected thoroughly at the time of exploration.

Finally, the amount of extravasation seen on cystography is related not only to the size of the laceration but also to the volume and rate of contrast infused; therefore, it cannot be used to determine the extent of the injury or the type of treatment.

Classification and incidence

Various published classifications of injuries to the urinary bladder exist [4], but at the 2002 Consensus Panel, four categories and incidences of injuries were agreed upon and are listed below [1].

Contusion (? %)
Intraperitoneal rupture (38%–40%)
Extraperitoneal rupture (54%–56%)
Combined intra- and extraperitoneal rupture (5%–8%)

Contusion

A true incidence of bladder contusions is difficult to convey as many minor lesions are silent clinically or the cystogram may be normal. This injury results from damage to the bladder mucosa and frequently the muscularis without loss of wall continuity. Extravasation cannot be seen but the bladder outline may be distorted.

Intraperitoneal rupture

When secondary to blunt trauma, this type of lesion is caused by a sudden increase in intravesical pressure that results in rupture of the dome, the weakest and most mobile part of the bladder. Contrast material fills the cul-de-sac, outlines loops of bowel, and extends into the paracolic gutter (Fig. 1).

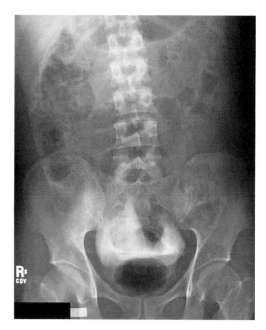

Fig. 1. Intraperitoneal bladder rupture. Postdrainage film from a conventional cystogram demonstrating contrast material outlining the paracolic gutter and between bowel loops indicative of intraperitoneal rupture.

Extraperitoneal rupture

This lesion is seen almost exclusively with pelvic fractures when caused by external violence [5]. As mentioned above, the shearing force of the attachments from the bladder to the bone as the ring is disrupted, or a bursting injury or puncture by a bone spicule, are the causes of these injuries. If there is a large pelvic hematoma, the bladder is compressed into a "teardrop deformity". Urinary extravasation may extend through the obturator foramen to the thigh, to the scrotum through the inguinal canal, or up the anterior abdominal wall or retroperitoneum (Fig. 2) [3].

Combined intra- and extraperitoneal rupture

These injuries are secondary to a pelvic fracture and penetrating trauma. The radiographic findings are a mixture of the previous descriptions of the single lesion (Fig. 3).

Therapy

Contusion

If marked hematuria exists, especially if clots are present, urethral catheter drainage with a large

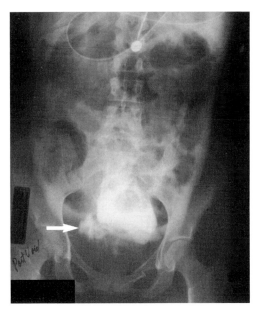

Fig. 3. Combined bladder rupture. Abdominal radiograph from a conventional cystogram demonstrates intraperitoneal and extraperitoneal (*arrow*) bladder rupture.

bore (22–24 French) Foley should be placed to straight drainage. Continuous bladder irrigation through a three-way catheter is discouraged for the outflow lumen in these catheters is small, which may prohibit clot evacuation. This could lead to catheter obstruction, bladder distention, and, possibly, bladder rupture at an area weakened by the traumatic event.

Catheter drainage also may be necessary if a large pelvic hematoma exists that is distorting the bladder or obstructing the bladder neck. Finally, patients who present with a sacral fracture may have neuropraxis as a result of nerve root damage and may be unable to urinate. When the catheter is removed in patients who present with a bladder contusion, they should be observed carefully until their voiding pattern returns to normal. Minor bladder contusions may not require catheter drainage if the patient is voiding to completion, but most of these patients are polytrauma victims and urine output monitoring is required for at least the first few days after injury [4,6].

Intraperitoneal rupture

When caused by blunt trauma to the full bladder, these lesions are usually large rents and

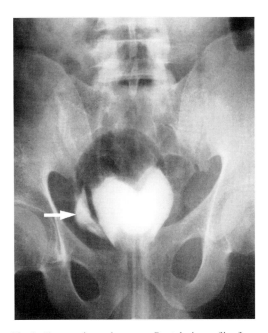

Fig. 2. Extraperitoneal rupture. Post-drainage film from a conventional cystogram demonstrates a flame-shaped area of contrast extravasation (*arrow*) from the right lateral aspect of the bladder characteristic of extraperitoneal rupture.

require immediate surgical repair. Usually, a two-layer watertight closure using absorbable suture is performed and the patient is left with a large bore urethral Foley catheter to straight drainage. Before closure, the interior of the bladder should be inspected for other injuries [13]. In the past, placement of a suprapubic tube was considered routine but rarely is this necessary [14]. Omit a suprapubic tube if a concomitant pelvic fracture is being repaired with internal metal plates to avoid a possible pelvic abscess.

If an iatrogenic penetrating injury occurs, is recognized immediately, is small, and the abdomen is soft and not distended, a large bore urethral Foley catheter may be placed to straight drainage and the patient observed and examined at frequent intervals. At the first sign of peritoneal irritation or distention or if the catheter fails to drain, a cystogram should be performed and immediate exploration considered depending on the findings.

A common emergency consultation to the operating room is from a surgeon performing some type of pelvic procedure who has realized the bladder has been entered. First, establish the extent of the injury by examining the entire organ, usually intravesically by enlarging the bladder wound. If the original surgeon has closed the bladder wound with sutures, remove them and perform a proper examination. Many times a second injury will be seen that was unrecognized when the obvious injury was discovered and repaired.

Penetrating injuries as a result of external violence, especially when caused by gunshot wounds, are handled best by surgical exploration and thorough inspection of the bladder with missile retrieval if possible. These patients commonly have multiple organs injured and exploration with careful examination of the missile tract and all abdominal organs is imperative.

Extraperitoneal rupture

If the only injury to the bladder is an extraperitoneal rupture, 10 days of catheter drainage allows the lesion to heal without surgical repair [3,6]; however, the catheter must have a large lumen and it must freely drain without the potential for obstruction with clots [15]. If the catheter does not drain properly or if the patient is going to have surgical exploration for another reason, formal surgical repair should be performed. Surgical repair is also mandatory if there is a concomitant vaginal or rectal injury or injury to the bladder neck [13,16].

The injury should be approached intravesically by opening the dome. The bladder must be inspected thoroughly and all tears closed with absorbable sutures. The bladder neck must be reconstructed and if the vagina is injured, it should be repaired at the same time [13,16]. A urethral catheter and, often, a suprapubic catheter are needed to obtain adequate drainage. The dome then is closed in two layers as described for an intraperitoneal injury.

Postoperative care

Antibiotics

Patients with indwelling Foley catheters eventually develop bacteruria even with closed system drainage. If treated with antibiotics, the chance that a resistant organism will colonize the patient is always there. If not treated until the catheter is removed, this threat is negligible.

Because most of these patients have multiple injuries and multiple physicians, they are almost always placed on antibiotics from the moment treatment is begun. A good compromise is to perform a urinalysis or a urine culture a month or two after the injury to be sure the urine is sterile.

Cystogram

Patients who have a contusion or a properly repaired intraperitoneal (dome) lesion should not need a cystogram. If the injury was a small iatrogenic intraperitoneal lesion, a cystogram should be performed before the catheter is removed, usually on the tenth day.

Patients who have extraperitoneal lesions as a result of external trauma treated by catheter drainage or formal repair need to have a cystogram on the tenth day before catheter removal. At least 85% of these lesions are healed by that time, but even with transvesical suturing, a watertight closure is never assured. The study should be repeated every 3 to 5 days after that if extravasation is present until it is no longer seen. Then the catheter can be removed and the patient observed until a return to normal voiding function occurs.

References

[1] Gomez R, Ceballos L, Coburn M, et al. Consensus statement on bladder injuries. BJU Int 2004;94(1): 27–32.

[2] Carroll P, McAninch J. Major bladder trauma. Mechanisms of injury and a unified method of diagnosis and repair. J Urol 1984;132:254–7.

[3] Corriere J, Sandler C. Mechanisms of injury, patterns of extravasation and management of extraperitoneal bladder rupture due to blunt trauma. J Urol 1988;139(1):43–4.

[4] Corriere JN Jr. Trauma to the lower urinary tract. In: Gillenwater JY, Grayhack JT, Howards SS, editors. Adult and pediatric urology. 4th edition. Philadelphia: Lippincott, Williams & Wilkins; 2002. p. 507–30.

[5] Palmer K, Benson G, Corriere J. Diagnosis and initial management of urologic injuries associated with 200 consecutive pelvic fractures. J Urol 1983;130(4):712–4.

[6] Corriere J, Sandler C. Management of the ruptured bladder: seven years of experience with 111 cases. J Urol 1986;126(3):830–3.

[7] Morey A, Iverson A, Swan A, et al. Bladder rupture after blunt trauma: guidelines for diagnostic imaging. J Trauma 2001;51(4):683–6.

[8] Corriere J, Sandler C. Bladder rupture from external trauma: diagnosis and management. World J Urol 1999;17:84–9.

[9] Haas C, Brown S, Spirnak J. Limitations of routine spiral computerized tomography in the evaluation of bladder trauma. J Urol 1999;162(1):51–2.

[10] Horstmann WG, McClennan BL, Heiken JP. Comparison of computed tomography and conventional cystography for detection of traumatic bladder rupture. Urol Radiol 1991;12:188–91.

[11] Peng M, Parisky Y, Cornwell E, et al. CT cystography versus conventional cystography in evaluation of bladder injury. Am J Roentgenol 1999;173(5):1269–72.

[12] Sandler C, Hall J, Rodriguez M, et al. Bladder injury in blunt pelvic trauma. Radiology 1986;158(3):633–8.

[13] Corriere JN Jr. Repair of traumatic bladder injuries. In: Libertino JA, editor. Reconstructive urologic surgery. 3rd edition. St. Louis (MO): Mosby; 1998. p. 241–5.

[14] Volpe M, Pachter E, Scalea T, et al. Is there a difference in outcome when treating traumatic intraperitoneal bladder rupture with or without a suprapubic tube? J Urol 1999;161(4):1103–5.

[15] Kotkin L, Koch M. Morbidity associated with nonoperative management of extraperitoneal bladder injuries. J Trauma 1995;38(6):895–8.

[16] Corriere JN Jr. Extraperitoneal bladder rupture. In: McAninch JW, editor. Traumatic and reconstructive urology. Philadelphia: WB Saunders; 1996. p. 269–73.

ELSEVIER
SAUNDERS

Urol Clin N Am 33 (2006) 73–85

UROLOGIC
CLINICS
of North America

Diagnosis and Classification of Urethral Injuries

Daniel I. Rosenstein, MD, FACS, FRCS (Urol)[a,b,*],
Nejd F. Alsikafi, MD[c,d]

[a]Division of Urology, Santa Clara Valley Medical Center, 751 South Bascom Avenue, San Jose, CA 95128, USA
[b]Department of Urology, Stanford University Medical Center, 300 Pasteur Drive, Stanford, CA 94305, USA
[c]Mount Sinai Medical Center, California Avenue at 15th Street, Chicago, IL 60608, USA
[d]Section of Urology, University of Chicago Medical Center, 5841 South Maryland Avenue, Chicago, IL 60637, USA

Urethral injuries arise from a variety of different insults, ranging from external violence to urethral instrumentation. Most result from blunt trauma, with penetrating injuries more commonly reported in the military setting [1]. The male urethra is anatomically subdivided into anterior and posterior segments at the level of the urogenital diaphragm, and mechanism of urethral injury may also be subclassified along these lines. Posterior urethral injury usually occurs in close proximity to the external (ie, voluntary) urethral sphincter mechanism, and is usually initiated by a massive shearing force that results in pelvic fracture and disruption through the membranous urethra [2]. Membranous urethral disruptions are associated with multiple organ injury, whereas anterior urethral injuries usually occur in isolation. Examples of anterior urethral injuries include straddle trauma crushing the immobile bulbous urethra against the pubic rami, or a rupture of the corporal bodies (eg, penile fracture), leading to a laceration through the adjacent urethra. Iatrogenic injuries affect both anterior and posterior segments of the urethra, and are increasingly frequent, possibly because of increasing numbers of transurethral procedures and radical prostatectomies.

A sound diagnostic acumen in dealing with urethral injuries includes a high index of suspicion, with avoidance of urethral catheter passage until a potential urethral injury has been excluded. Certain clinical signs and symptoms will point the clinician toward a possible urethral injury, with a properly performed radiographic study confirming the diagnosis. Once the presence of a urethral injury has been diagnosed, the injury may be subclassified according to well-defined radiographic findings. These findings, as well as the overall condition of the patient, will in turn guide judicious initial management of the injured urethra.

This article concentrates on reviewing the major etiologies and mechanisms of urethral injury. For purposes of convenience and clarity, posterior and anterior urethral injuries due to external trauma are presented separately. The article discusses both clinical diagnostic findings and radiographic studies for each type of injury, and reviews the classification systems commonly used in urethral trauma. Iatrogenic urethral injuries, which may affect both anterior and posterior urethra, are reviewed separately. Female urethral injuries are also discussed. Timely and accurate diagnosis of urethral injuries leads to appropriate acute management and reduces long-term morbidity.

Anatomy

Understanding urethral injuries begins with a detailed comprehension of urethral anatomy. The adult male urethra is approximately 18 cm long, with the posterior urethra comprising the proximal 3 cm, and the anterior urethra comprising the remaining 15 cm, with the division point

* Corresponding author. Santa Clara Valley Medical Center, Physician's Annex, 751 South Bascom Avenue, San Jose, California 95128.

E-mail address: Daniel.Rosenstein@hhs.co.santa-clara.ca.us (D.I. Rosenstein).

between the two located at the perineal membrane. The urethra may be further subdivided into five segments (Fig. 1):

Posterior urethra:
- Prostatic urethra
- Membranous urethra

Anterior urethra:
- Bulbous urethra
- Pendulous urethra
- Fossa navicularis [3]

The posterior urethra begins as the prostatic urethra at the level of the bladder neck and extends as a channel through the prostate, anterior to the midline. The bladder neck (ie, internal) sphincter extends from the internal meatus through the prostatic urethra to the level of the verumontanum. This sphincter is comprised most proximally of circular fibers of smooth muscle, which provide passive continence via tonic sympathetic fiber activity.

The prostatic urethra ends distal to the verumontanum, which is a 0.5 cm long protuberance found on the ventral wall of the urethra. The paired ejaculatory ducts empty into the prostatic urethra at the level of the verumontanum. The prostate itself is located deep within the pelvis, and is closely adherent to the posterior aspect of

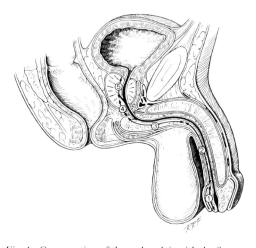

Fig. 1. Cross section of the male pelvis with the five urethral segments labeled. (1) Fossa navicularis. (2) Pendulous urethra. (3) Bulbous urethra. (4) Membranous urethra. (5) Prostatic urethra. (From Jordan GH, Schellhammer PF. Urethral surgery and stricture disease. In: Droller M, editor. Surgical management of urologic disease. St. Louis (MO): Mosby-Yearbook; 1992. p. 394.)

the anterior pubic arch at the level of the paired puboprostatic ligaments.

The membranous urethra is approximately 1 to 1.5 cm long, extending between the prostatic apex and the proximal corpus spongiosum. The membranous urethra is the only segment of the urethra that is unprotected by surrounding spongy tissue or prostatic stroma, and is thus more susceptible to external trauma. The distal sphincter mechanism is a combined voluntary and involuntary unit, with an outer layer of striated muscle fibers and an inner layer of smooth muscle intrinsic to the urethral wall [4]. The distal sphincter mechanism is typically about 2 cm long, but only 3 to 5 mm thick. Supporting the distal sphincter mechanism is an extrinsic periurethral striated muscle, which is under voluntary control. Contrary to early descriptions, the urogenital diaphragm does not completely encircle the membranous urethra, but rather forms an incomplete sling that offers posterior and lateral support. While each sphincteric unit may independently maintain passive continence once its confrere has been injured, the striated periurethral muscle may only assist with active continence (eg, interruption of voiding).

The bulbous urethra commences proximally at the level of the inferior aspect of the urogenital diaphragm, where it pierces and courses through the corpus spongiosum. The corpus spongiosum is a highly vascular network of elastic and smooth muscle fibers. A fibrous capsule known as the tunica albuginea surrounds the corpus spongiosum. The corpus spongiosum and the corpora cavernosa are in turn enclosed by two successive fascial layers. These layers are Buck's fascia and dartos fascia. Buck's fascia is the denser of the two layers, and is itself composed of an inner and outer lamina. The two laminae of Buck's fascia split to enclose the corpus spongiosum. The dartos fascia is a loose subdermal connective tissue layer that is continuous with the Colles' fascia in the perineum.

The urethral lumen remains eccentrically dorsally positioned in the corpus spongiosum throughout the bulbous urethra, but is centrally located in the pendulous urethra. The bulbous urethra is by definition enclosed not only by the corpus spongiosum, but also by the midline fusion of the ischiocavernosus (ie, bulbospongiosus) musculature. The bulbospongiosus muscle terminates just proximal to the penoscrotal junction, where the urethra continues distally as the pendulous urethra. The pendulous urethra is closely adherent to the corporal bodies dorsally. The distal most portion of the anterior urethra is the fossa navicularis, which is surrounded by the spongy tissue of the glans penis.

The adult female urethra is approximately 4 cm long, and extends from the urethrovesical junction at the bladder neck to the vaginal vestibule. Two layers of smooth muscle that extend distally from the bladder neck encircle the proximal part of the urethra. The inner layer is circular, whereas the outer layer runs longitudinally. The smooth muscle is further surrounded by a striated muscle layer (ie, rhabdosphincter), which is thickest at the level of the mid-urethra, and relatively deficient at its posterior aspect (Fig. 2) [4].

Traumatic posterior urethral injuries

Etiology

Blunt trauma causes the vast majority of injuries to the posterior urethra. Historically, many of these injuries were associated with industrial or mining accidents [5]. However, improvements in industrial safety and the rise of the automobile have shifted the etiology of these injuries, leading to a decline in such injuries related to industrial accidents and a rise in injuries related to motor-vehicle mishaps. Urethral disruption occurs in approximately 10% of pelvic

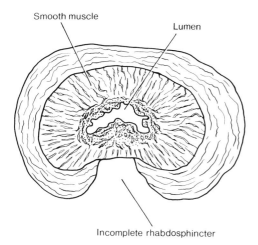

Fig. 2. The female urethra as seen in cross section. The rhabdosphincter is incomplete posteriorly. (*From* Mac-Diarmid SA, Chapple CR. Surgical management of injuries to the bladder neck. In: McAninch JW, editor. Traumatic and reconstructive urology. Philadelphia: W.B. Saunders; 1996. p. 539.)

fractures, but almost all membranous urethral disruptions related to blunt trauma have an associated pelvic fracture [6]. The pelvic fractures that lead to urethral disruption are usually secondary to motor-vehicle accidents (68%–84%) or falls from heights and pelvic crush injuries (6%–25%) [7]. Pedestrians are far more at risk than passengers of suffering pelvic-fracture urethral-disruption injuries in motor-vehicle accidents. Other unusual causes of pelvic fracture and membranous urethral injury include horse kicks to the perineum [8] and injuries related to mechanical bulls (ie, the "urban cowboy" syndrome) [9].

Pelvic fractures occur predominantly in the first three decades of life, with a male/female ratio of 2:1 in young adults [10]. Furthermore, urethral injuries associated with pelvic fractures are much less common in females [11]. Some authorities have postulated that the female urethra is at a lower risk of injury because of its shorter length and its greater mobility in relation to the pubic arch [12]. Although pelvic fracture urethral injuries are rare in females overall, they predominate in the prepubertal and pubescent age groups. This tendency is likely because younger females have thinner and less mobile urethral tissues, and have compressible pelvic bones [13].

Because the forces causing pelvic crush injury leading to urethral disruption may be extreme, nonurologic injuries are frequently associated with pelvic fractures. In fact, such injuries are far more frequent than urethral injuries. These nonurologic injuries, including head or spinal-cord trauma, respiratory and musculoskeletal injuries, take precedence in the initial resuscitation of the multiply injured trauma victim [10]. Bladder rupture occurs in approximately 5% to 10% of pelvic fractures. With an associated urethral injury, the rate increases to 10% to 20% [14]. This associated urethral injury is most commonly an extraperitoneal rupture (56%–78%), but may be an intraperitoneal rupture (17%–39%), and least commonly a combined intra- and extraperitoneal rupture [15]. Concomitant injury to the bladder neck may have particularly devastating consequences in terms of continence. Because of the high association of urethral disruption with bladder rupture, all such patients require cystography to investigate this possibility. Prepubertal males are more likely to suffer extension of the disruption up into and through the prostatic urethra. This increased vulnerability to such injury is likely because the prostate is smaller and less protective at that age [8].

Female urethral injuries frequently have associated vaginal lacerations and concomitant rectal tears. In his recent series of pelvic-fracture-related injuries of the female urethra, Mundy reported a 75% incidence of vaginal injury and a 33% incidence of rectal injury [16].

Pelvic fractures: subtypes and risk stratification

Pelvic fractures may be classified according to the direction of the major force of injury, including lateral compression, anteroposterior compression, and vertical shear injuries [17]. In 1987, Young and Burgess first described this classification, which has been useful for orthopedic surgeons for prognosticating blood loss, deformity reduction, and fixation, among other variables [18]. Anteroposterior compression injuries are associated with an increased incidence of abdominal visceral and pelvic vascular injuries. These injuries open the pelvis and major morbidity results from pelvic bleeding. Lateral compression injuries, which close the pelvis, account for the largest number of associated injuries and complications of pelvic fractures [19]. Vertical shear injuries usually result from falls from great heights or from posterior forces applied to a fixed pelvis. These fractures cause disruption of both the anterior and posterior pelvic complexes, with the fractured hemipelvis moving separately from the opposite side. Pelvic fractures may also be classified as clinically stable or unstable. Vertical shear injuries are grossly unstable, while anteroposterior and lateral compression injuries are more commonly stable [18].

For the purposes of the urologist suspicious of urethral injury, certain pelvic fracture subtypes have a higher association with urethral disruption [20]. These subtypes include straddle fractures, which are also called butterfly fractures, where all four pubic rami are fractured. Another subtype is the Malgaigne fracture, involving disruption through ischiopubic rami anteriorly as well as through the sacrum or sacroiliac joint posteriorly. In a prospective study assessing the risk ratio of pelvic fracture subtype to membranous urethral injury, Koraitim found the highest risk for straddle fracture, with an odds ratio of 3.85, and Malgaigne fracture, with an odds ratio of 3.40 [7]. If a straddle fracture is combined with a sacroiliac joint diastasis, the odds ratio increases to 24.02 [7]. Conversely, the risk of urethral injury in fractures not involving the ischiopubic rami is negligible.

Pelvic fractures may thus be classified as low or high risk in terms of associated urethral disruption. The information obtained from initial pelvic radiography should be combined with clinical data in evaluating urethral injuries. In a recent retrospective study of 43 patients with lower urologic injuries in the context of pelvic fractures, Ziran found 10 patients whose injuries were missed at the initial evaluation [21]. Three patients in this series had missed urethral disruptions, which were ultimately discovered at the time of urgent exploratory laparotomy. All 3 patients in this subgroup had no clinical findings suggestive of urethral disruption (ie, no blood at the meatus and normal digital rectal exam). Nonetheless, all 3 patients had pelvic fractures at high risk for urethral disruption (ie, 2 had straddle plus sacral ala fracture, and 1 had a Malgaigne fracture). Radiographic findings on the initial anteroposterior pelvic film may thus rarely be the only clues suggesting urethral injury.

Mechanism of injury

The traditional concept of the mechanism of prostatomembranous urethral disruption involves a shearing force that avulses the apex of the prostate from the membranous urethra [22], where the membranous urethra is fixed in place by the urogenital diaphragm. Because the initial injury lacerates through the distal sphincter mechanism at the level of the membranous urethra, any future continence depends upon a competent bladder neck sphincter [23]. Pokorny postulated three mechanisms through which this shearing may occur [24]. The first involves upward displacement of one hemipelvis and symphysis (eg, in a Malgaigne fracture), with laceration into the urethra. The second mechanism includes straddle fractures whereby a free floating central symphyseal fragment is displaced posteriorly, leading to disruption. The third mechanism involves pubic symphysis diastasis, whereby the membranous urethra is stretched until it ruptures.

However, this traditional mechanism of injury has recently been called into question [25]. A number of studies have undermined this view, including Mundy's recent work, which attempted to prospectively study distal urethral sphincter function following anastomotic repair of a pelvic-fracture urethral-disruption defect [26]. Most the 20 subjects in this study showed endoscopic and urodynamic evidence of distal sphincter function. Although this study provides indirect evidence of distal sphincter function and injury distal to the external sphincter, more convincing direct anatomic support for this view has come from a recent cadaveric study by Mouraviev and Santucci [27]. In this dissection study of victims who died with known pelvic-fracture urethral-disruption injuries, seven out of 10 subjects were found to have disruption distal to the external urinary sphincter. This evidence suggests that urethral disruption more likely represents partial or complete avulsion of the membranous urethra off the fixed bulbous urethra at the bulbomembranous junction.

Diagnosis of posterior urethral injury: clinical aspects

The possibility of posterior urethral injury should be suspected in the presence of a suspected or confirmed pelvic fracture. As noted previously, certain pelvic fracture subtypes are more likely associated with urethral disruption. Blood at the meatus is a cardinal sign of posterior urethral injury, and is seen in 37% to 93% of cases [28]. However, the amount of blood at the meatus does not appear to correlate with the severity of the injury [29]. A palpably distended bladder or inability to void, perineal bruising, and perineal ecchymosis are all suggestive of urethral disruption [30]. Digital rectal exam may disclose an elevated or displaced prostate gland in 34% of cases [31], but may be impalpable secondary to the significant hematoma that surrounds the prostate in the setting of pelvic fracture. Digital rectal exam may also disclose blood on the examining finger, which is highly suggestive of a rectal injury [6]. The triad of pelvic fracture, blood at the meatus, and inability to void are diagnostic of prostato-membranous urethral disruption [32].

Before the advent of widespread retrograde urethrography, unsuccessful catheterization attempts in pelvic-fracture patients were considered diagnostic of urethral disruption. Today, in the era of urethrography, the practice of attempting to catheterize pelvic-fracture patients should be condemned. However, the practice continues. A recent study of patients with suspected urethral disruption found 11 of 57 (19.3%) patients with catheters placed outside the bladder before arrival at the emergency room [33].

Unfortunately, none of the clinical findings listed above is entirely reliable in diagnosing a urethral disruption. Most urologists have argued that urethral catheterization attempts in the presence of the findings discussed above are contraindicated before diagnostic retrograde urethrography [32]. Those who support this argument cite the possibility of infecting the pelvic hematoma, as well as potentially converting a partial urethral rupture to a complete tear [34]. They also argue that such catheterization will result in inadequate staging of the injury. Others familiar with such issues argue that a single gentle attempt at catheterization is unlikely to create permanent damage. They also point out that, if the catheterization is unsuccessful, the attempt can be immediately followed by retrograde urethrography [10]. Urologists have debated this controversial point for several decades. All urologists would agree that the diagnostic study of choice is retrograde urethrography, and the threshold for performing it in the setting of suspected urethral injury should be low. Occasionally, a critically injured and unstable patient may require urgent bladder drainage before retrograde urethrography. In this case, the most prudent and expedient approach is to insert a percutaneous suprapubic catheter and evaluate the urethra once the patient is more stable [35].

Diagnosis of posterior urethral injury: radiographic aspects

Retrograde urethrography has become the study of choice in diagnosing urethral injuries. It is accurate, simple, and may be performed rapidly in the trauma setting [36]. While CT scanning is ideal for imaging upper urinary tract and bladder injuries, it has a limited role in the diagnosis of urethral injuries [37]. Nonetheless, a recent retrospective radiographic comparison of CT findings in patients with urethrographically proven urethral injuries revisited this issue [38]. Ali demonstrated CT findings of prostatic apex elevation and contrast extravasation above or below the urogenital diaphragm in various subclasses of urethral injury. While MRI is useful for imaging the posttraumatic pelvis before reconstruction [39], this modality has no role in urethral imaging in the trauma setting. Similarly, urethral ultrasound has limited diagnostic use in the acute setting. Ultrasonography may be useful in localizing the pelvic hematoma and bladder for planned suprapubic catheter placement.

Retrograde urethrography begins with proper patient positioning on the x-ray table. The patient should be supine with the pelvis elevated to 30° to 45° oblique to the horizontal plane. The thigh closest to the table is flexed 90°, whereas the upper thigh is kept straight. This position allows clear visualization of the entire urethra, and should prevent the pelvic bones from obscuring any extravasation (Fig. 3). A scout film should be obtained to confirm correct positioning before urethrography. Oblique positioning may be limited by discomfort related to pelvic fractures.

The simplest technique of urethrography involves insertion of a 60 cc catheter tip syringe into the meatus for contrast injection. However, this method is discouraged because it results in unnecessary radiation of the operator's hand. Ideally, a 14 Fr Foley catheter is inserted into the fossa navicularis with the balloon inflated to 2 cc to seat the tip and prevent contrast from refluxing out the meatus. The catheter is then connected to a 60 cc catheter tip syringe filled with water-soluble undiluted contrast material. Then 30 cc of contrast material is injected retrograde into the urethra, with a single radiograph exposure taken toward the end of injection. This method permits adequate distension of the urethra, and should permit visualization of any extravasated contrast material. Fluoroscopic guidance during the study is ideal but is not absolutely necessary for diagnostic purposes.

In a retrograde urethrogram of an uninjured urethra, a smooth and continuous contour will be seen through the bulbous urethra. The contour typically cones down at the bulbomembranous junction. The normal prostatic urethra appears as a narrow passage with visible indentation by the verumontanum. An adequate retrograde urethrogram includes a jet of contrast passing through the bladder neck into the bladder (Fig. 4). Abnormalities on urethrography are readily identified and may be classified as outlined in the following section.

Classification of posterior urethral injuries

The most common classification system currently in use for blunt posterior urethral injuries was described by Colapinto and McCallum in 1977 [29]. Goldman and colleagues recently modified the system to include all common types of blunt urethral injuries [40]. This classification uses radiographic findings to sort blunt urethral injuries by type:

Type 1: Rupture of the puboprostatic ligaments and surrounding periprostatic hematoma stretch the membranous urethra without rupture (Fig. 5A).

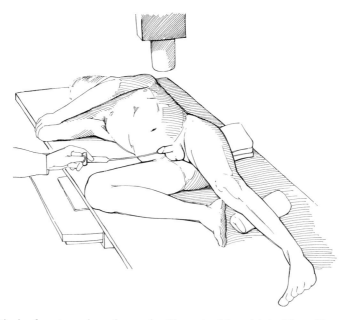

Fig. 3. Correct positioning for retrograde urethrography. The angle of the pelvis is oblique. The examiner's hand is kept away from the x-ray beam. (*From* Armenakas NA, McAninch JW. Acute anterior urethral injuries: diagnosis and initial management. In: McAninch JW, editor. Traumatic and reconstructive urology. Philadelphia: W.B. Saunders; 1996. p. 547.)

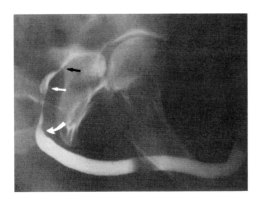

Fig. 4. A normal retrograde urethrogram. The anterior urethra has a smooth contour. Curved arrow shows where the normal bulbous urethra terminates at the cone-shaped bulbomembranous junction. The straight white arrow shows the verumontanum within the prostatic urethra. Contrast may be seen emanating into the bladder through the bladder neck at the level of the black arrow. (*From* Rosen MA, McAninch JW. Preoperative staging of the anterior urethral stricture. In: McAninch JW, editor. Traumatic and reconstructive urology. Philadelphia: W.B. Saunders; 1996. p. 552.)

Type 2: Partial or complete rupture of the membranous urethra above the urogenital diaphragm or perineal membrane. On urethrography, contrast material is seen extravasating above the perineal membrane into the pelvis (Fig. 5B).

Type 3: Partial or complete rupture of the membranous urethra with disruption of the urogenital diaphragm. Contrast extravasates both into the pelvis and out into the perineum (Fig. 5C).

Type 4: Bladder neck injury with extension into the urethra.

Type 4a: Extraperitoneal bladder rupture at the bladder base with periurethral extravasation, simulating a Type 4 injury.

Type 5: Pure anterior urethral injury.

Type 1 and 2 injuries are uncommon, each representing approximately 10% to 15% of posterior urethral injuries [41]. Either Type 2 or Type 3 injuries may be classified as complete or partial ruptures. The relative incidence of complete to partial tears is approximately 3:1 [20]. This radiographic distinction is clinically significant because partial tears may heal without significant stricture formation, whereas complete tears rarely do. Type 3 injuries are the most frequent, occurring in 66% to 85% of all cases [20]. Type 4 injuries are rare,

but may have potentially dire consequences in terms of continence if they go unrecognized. Using radiographic appearance alone to distinguish Type 4 from Type 4a injuries may be difficult.

Another classification system for pelvic-fracture urethral injuries was recently introduced by Al Rifaei [42]. This classification system adds subcategories for proximal prostatic avulsion and attempts to distinguish injuries based upon evaluation of the sphincteric mechanism. This classification system has not yet been widely accepted.

Traumatic anterior urethral injury

Etiology and mechanism

Blunt or penetrating trauma may cause anterior urethral injuries. Blunt injuries are more commonly diagnosed, and the bulbous urethra is the most frequently injured segment (85%) [43] because it is fixed beneath the pubic bone, unlike the freely mobile pendulous urethra. Blunt injuries to the bulbous urethra are typically caused by straddle type injuries (eg, motor-vehicle accidents; bicycle accidents; falling astride onto a fence, railing or saddle) or kicks to the perineum. The force contacting the perineum crushes the bulbous urethra up against the inferior pubic rami, leading to contusion or urethral laceration [44] (Fig. 6).

Unlike prostatomembranous urethral disruptions, blunt anterior urethral trauma rarely has significant associated organ trauma. In fact, the straddle injury may be mild enough that the patient seeks no treatment at the time of the acute event. These patients typically present with bulbar urethral strictures after an interval of months to years [45]. In the recent review of straddle injuries to the bulbar urethra by Park and McAninch, 47 of 78 patients (60%) presented 6 months to 10 years after the acute injury with obstructive voiding symptoms or frank urinary retention [46].

Traumatic anterior urethral disruptions may also be related to penile fracture in 10% to 20% of cases. The mechanism of injury is typically a direct blow or buckling force applied to the erect penis during intercourse, with the erect penis striking the female pubic ramus. This force tears the tunica albuginea and leads to rapid detumescence and pain.

If the tear in the tunica extends into the corpus spongiosum, a urethral injury may result. Most patients are able to urinate normally following penile fracture, but the urologist must maintain a high index of suspicion for urethral injury.

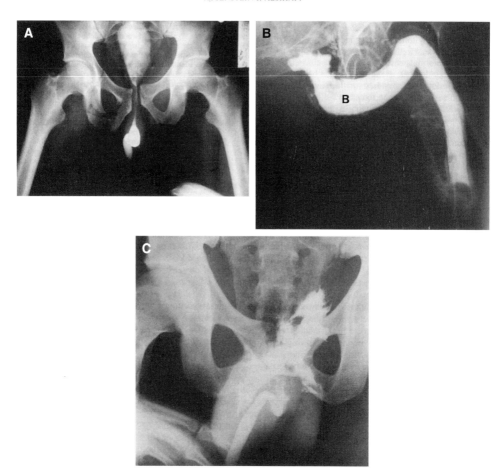

Fig. 5. Prostatomembranous urethral disruption injuries. (*A*) Type 1: Membranous urethra is stretched without rupture. Note the "pear shaped" bladder as a result of compression by perivesical hemorrhage. (*B*) Type 2: Complete rupture of the membranous urethra with intact urogenital diaphragm. Extravasation extends into the pelvis only. (*C*) Type 3: Complete rupture of the membranous urethra with disrupted urogenital diaphragm and injury to the proximal bulbous urethra. Extravasation extends into the pelvis as well as into the perineum. (*From* Dixon CM. Diagnosis and acute management of posterior urethral disruptions. In: McAninch JW, editor. Traumatic and reconstructive urology. Philadelphia: W.B. Saunders; 1996. p. 350.)

Failure to void spontaneously may signify compression of the urethra by hematoma but should lead to evaluation of urethral injury by retrograde urethrography. Urethral injury occurs in up to one third of cases and usually consists of partial disruption, although complete transection can result. Retrograde urethrography is mandatory in all patients with blood at the urethral meatus, hematuria of any extent, or inability to void [47].

Penetrating trauma to the urethra is most often caused by firearms, but can also result from stab wounds, industrial accidents, self-mutilation attempts, and bites. In all cases, general principles of management include judicious debridement and

hemostasis within the wound, as well as careful exploration and repair of corporal and urethral injuries. Most civilian penile gunshot wounds are caused by low-velocity missiles, which cause damage only in the path of the bullet. Associated wounds of the thigh and pelvis are common, and may require urgent exploration and repair [47].

Urethral injury is determined by careful physical examination, with special attention paid to the trajectory of the bullet and initial hemostasis. The finding of a palpable corporeal defect in combination with an expanding penile hematoma or significant bleeding from the entry and exit wounds is highly predictive of corporeal injury,

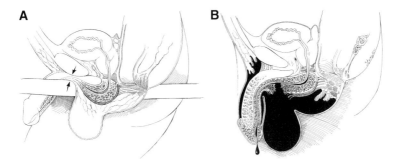

Fig. 6. Mechanism of blunt anterior urethral trauma. (*A*) Straddle injury illustrating the bulbous urethra crushed against the pubic symphysis. (*B*) Resulting urethral disruption with hemorrhage extending along the confines of Colles' fascia. Buck's fascia has been disrupted. (*From* Armenakas NA, McAninch JW. Acute anterior urethral injuries: diagnosis and initial management. In: McAninch JW, editor. Traumatic and reconstructive urology. Philadelphia: W.B. Saunders; 1996. p. 545.)

and should prompt expedient exploration [48]. Urethral injury, which occurs in 25% to 40% of penetrating injuries to the penis, should be excluded with retrograde urethrography in all cases [49]. The bullet may directly lacerate the urethra, or result in urethral injury via delayed necrosis of adjacent spongy tissue. The triad of no blood at the meatus, absence of hematuria, and normal voiding suggests that no urethral injury has occurred.

Penile amputation is an unusual cause of penetrating urethral injury, typically resulting from attempts at self-emasculation in the actively psychotic patient. Penile amputation has also been reported as a rare but devastating complication of circumcision.

Penetrating anterior urethral trauma may be caused by insertion of foreign bodies into the urethra because of mental illness or for autoerotic purposes [50]. In their recent review of a 17-year single-center experience with urethral foreign bodies, Rahman, Elliott, and McAninch reported the most common symptom to be dysuria and frequency. The foreign body was palpable in all patients, and plain images were sufficient to diagnose the location and shape of most of the foreign bodies [51]. Endoscopic retrieval was successful in most cases.

Diagnosis

The presence of an anterior urethral injury is frequently suggested by the history, as outlined above. Any patient with recent blunt or penetrating trauma to the perineum, genitalia, or pelvis should be suspected of harboring a urethral injury [43]. Diagnosis may be delayed in some patients (eg, those with penile fractures, foreign bodies,

penile constriction bands) because of embarrassment. Significant delays in diagnosis with massive urinary extravasation may result in sepsis and severe (ie, necrotizing) infection [32]. This presentation may include swelling, discoloration and frank necrosis of the overlying perineal and genital skin.

In the case of penetrating trauma, the type of weapon used and the size and trajectory of the missile or knife are important historical clues. A voiding history, including ability to void, presence of dysuria, and time of last micturition, should be obtained. If available, a voided specimen should be analyzed for the presence of hematuria.

Blood at the meatus is once again the cardinal sign of anterior urethral injury [2]. Dysuria, hematuria, and inability to void are all strongly suggestive of urethral injury. A significant perineal hematoma will be present if the injury has disrupted Buck's fascia and tracks deep to Colles' fascia, creating a characteristic "butterfly" hematoma in the perineum [52]. This occurs in severe straddle injuries. Conversely, the hematoma remains contained in a sleeve distribution along the penile shaft if Buck's fascia remains intact. The urethra may rarely be completely extruded through the genital skin, indicative of complete disruption [53].

Radiographic staging with retrograde urethrography is conducted as described previously. Once again, no attempts at catheterization or voiding should be instituted until the urethral injury has been properly and completely staged.

Classification

The most widely used classification system for anterior urethral injuries was described by

McAninch and Armenakas [44] and is based upon radiographic findings:

1. Contusion: Clinical features suggest urethral injury, but retrograde urethrography is normal.
2. Incomplete disruption: Urethrography demonstrates extravasation, but urethral continuity is partially maintained. Contrast is seen filling the proximal urethra or bladder (Fig. 7).
3. Complete disruption: Urethrography demonstrates extravasation with absent filling of the proximal urethra or bladder. Urethral continuity is disrupted.

Iatrogenic urethral injury

Iatrogenic urethral injuries most commonly result from prolonged or traumatic urethral instrumentation, whereby the delicate mucosa may be partially disrupted. Denudation of the urethral mucosa exposes the underlying vascular spongy tissue to the passage of urine. The inflammatory cascade thus initiated leads to spongiofibrosis, which is scarring within the corpus spongiosum. The clinical manifestation of spongiofibrosis is urethral stricture disease. Most iatrogenic injuries in the anterior urethra occur within the bulbous urethra.

The most frequent cause of acute iatrogenic urethral trauma is related to traumatic Foley

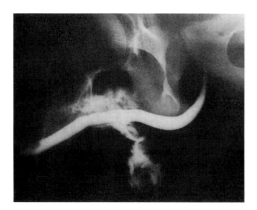

Fig. 7. Retrograde urethrogram demonstrating incomplete disruption of the anterior urethra secondary to a gunshot wound. Note contrast extravasation inferiorly and superiorly into adjacent corporal tissue. (*From* Miller KS, McAninch JW. Penile fracture and soft tissue injury. In: McAninch JW, editor. Traumatic and reconstructive urology. Philadelphia: W.B. Saunders; 1996. p. 697.)

catheter removal without prior balloon deflation. These injuries usually result in minor contusions that heal with few sequelae. Chronic indwelling urethral catheters generate prolonged inflammation and pressure necrosis of the urethral mucosa, leading to infection, erosion, and stricture disease. Changes in catheter design, specifically the introduction of less irritative silicone catheters, may have reduced the incidence of this injury.

Intermittent catheterization has a lower incidence of urethral injury when compared with indwelling urethral catheters. Hydrophilic coated catheters have a reduced incidence of urethral trauma and inflammation when compared with non-hydrophilic coated catheters [54] when used for intermittent catheterization.

Various treatments for urethral stricture disease may lead to further urethral injury. Repeated dilations and urethrotomies for stricture disease establish a chronic inflammatory process, which is perpetuated by further urine extravasation and scarring. Barbagli performed histological analysis on posturethrotomy urethral segments that were excised at the time of urethroplasty, and found diffuse inflammation throughout the corpus spongiosum [55]. While the UroLume endoprosthesis has occasionally been used successfully in the treatment of short bulbar strictures, it may also cause further urethral injury and lead to complete obstruction with fibrosis or intrastent hyperplastic response [56].

Urethral injuries have also been attributed to complications of extracorporeal circulation during cardiac revascularization surgery. Perioperative urethral catheterization has been implicated, and a recent retrospective analysis revealed a 6.6% stricture rate compared with 0% for a comparable group with suprapubic urinary drainage [57]. It has been hypothesized that urethral ischemia during extracorporeal circulation causes the injury [58]. In examining this problem, Bamshad recently demonstrated a significant decrease in intraoperative urethral blood flow using laser Doppler flowmetry during cardiopulmonary bypass [59].

Urethral injuries have also been recently reported as a complication of bladder-drained pancreas transplantation and pancreas-kidney transplantation [60]. This complication stems from pancreatic enzymes, which cause mucosal irritation. The injury may range from minor contusion to complete disruption with urinary extravasation [61].

Iatrogenic injuries of the posterior urethra have largely resulted from treatments for benign prostatic hyperplasia (BPH) as well as those for prostate cancer. These injuries frequently manifest themselves as urethral strictures at variable intervals following the initial treatment. While the term "posterior urethral stricture" has been used to encompass both pelvic-fracture prostatomembranous urethral disruptions and strictures within the posterior urethra following iatrogenic trauma, the term is a misnomer. In the case of pelvic-fracture prostatomembranous urethral disruptions, the urethra is not strictured, but rather its continuity is disrupted by intervening scar tissue. In the case of strictures within the posterior urethra following iatrogenic trauma, the urethra remains in continuity with a stenotic lumen. To highlight this distinction, the Société Internationale d'Urologie recently recommended that membranous urethral strictures occurring after transurethral prostate resection (TURP) or radical prostatectomy be referred to as "sphincter stenoses" [30].

Anastomotic urethral stricture following radical retropubic prostatectomy occurs in 7% to 17% of patients [62]. The risk increases with prior external beam radiation, as well as any factor that causes anastomotic ischemia (eg, microvascular disease, hypertension) or prolonged anastomotic extravasation [63]. Urethral strictures following TURP occur in 3.1% to 10% of patients [62,64]. Possible causes include postoperative urinary tract infection, urethral abrasion secondary to oversized resectoscopes, and current leakage through the sheath, leading to electrical urethral burn [65].

Urethral injury also occurs during minimally invasive procedures for BPH. A recent review reported on three patients who developed symptomatic mid-prostatic-urethral strictures following transurethral microwave therapy (TUMT) [66]. The investigators postulate that TUMT causes direct thermal or ischemic damage to the urethra despite continuous urethral cooling.

Female urethral injuries

Female urethral injury secondary to trauma is rare, but has been described in association with pelvic fracture in as many as 6% of cases [67]. The injury is usually associated with a vaginal laceration, which is the most frequent clue in reaching the diagnosis. Labial edema, hematuria, and urethrorrhagia may also be present. Unfortunately, these injuries are frequently missed because a vaginal exam is omitted in these severely injured patients.

Imaging of the female urethra in the case of suspected disruption may be difficult. Retrograde urethrography is technically challenging in this setting, and may reveal varying degrees of contrast extravasation and bladder compression by pelvic hematoma. McAninch has suggested that females with suspected urethral injury undergo diagnostic urethroscopy [68].

From a mechanistic standpoint, these injuries present as an anterior longitudinal urethral tear of varying length extending down from the bladder neck into the urethra [69], or as a partial or complete urethral avulsion. Perry and Husmann described 5 patients with longitudinal lacerations in 1992 [69]. In Mundy's recently published series of 12 patients [16], 5 had longitudinal tears, and 7 had complete urethral avulsion injuries. He suggests that avulsion injuries are likely secondary to more severe injury. Because these injuries are rare, a classification system and accepted guidelines for therapy have yet to be formally established.

Summary

Urethral injury originates from a number of well-defined etiologies, as outlined here. Recognition of cardinal signs and symptoms of urethral injury facilitates timely radiographic diagnosis and classification in most cases. This information may then permit appropriate initial management. The astute clinician must maintain a high index of suspicion, as these injuries are both uncommon and frequently overshadowed by multisystem trauma. Although the injury may assume secondary importance in the acute trauma setting, failure to accurately diagnose urethral injuries may lead to sequelae (eg, stricture disease, incontinence, erectile dysfunction), which linger long after other injuries have disappeared.

References

[1] Herr HW, McAninch JW. Urethral injuries in the Civil War. J Urol 2005;173:1090–3.

[2] McAninch JW. Traumatic injuries to the urethra. J Trauma 1981;21:291–7.

[3] Jordan GH. Management of membranous urethral distraction injuries via the perineal approach. In: McAninch JW, Jordan GH, Carroll PR, editors. Traumatic and reconstructive urology. Philadelphia: W.B. Saunders; 1996. p. 393.

[4] MacDiarmid SA, Chapple CR. Surgical management of injuries to the bladder neck. In: McAninch JW, Jordan GH, Carroll PR, editors. Traumatic and

reconstructive urology. Philadelphia: W.B. Saunders; 1996. p. 533–40.

[5] Kaiser TF, Farrow FC. Injury to the bladder and prostatomembranous urethra associated with fracture of the bony pelvis. Surg Gynecol Obstet 1965; 120:99.

[6] Palmer JK, Benson GS, Corriere JN. Diagnosis and initial management of urological injuries associated with 200 consecutive pelvic fractures. J Urol 1983; 130:712–4.

[7] Koraitim MM, Marzouk ME, Atta MA, et al. Risk factors and mechanism of urethral injury in pelvic fractures. Br J Urol 1996;71:876.

[8] Koraitim MM. Post-traumatic posterior urethral strictures in children: a 20 year experience. J Urol 1997;157:641.

[9] Green RS, Maier R. The urban cowboy syndrome revisited: case report. South Med J 2003;96(12): 1262–4.

[10] Mundy AR. Pelvic fracture injuries of the posterior urethra. World J Urol 1999;17:90–5.

[11] Antoci SP, Schiff M. Bladder and urethral injuries in patients with pelvic fractures. J Urol 1982;128:25.

[12] Chapple CR. Urethral injury. BJU Int 2000;86: 318–26.

[13] Hemal AK, Dorairajan LN, Gupta NP. Post-traumatic complete and partial loss of urethra with pelvic fracture in girls. An appraisal of management. J Urol 2000;163:282–7.

[14] Corriere JN, Sandler CM. Mechanisms of injury, patterns of extravasation and management of extraperitoneal bladder rupture secondary to blunt trauma. J Urol 1988;139:43–4.

[15] Carlin BI, Resnick MI. Indications and techniques for urologic evaluation of the trauma patient with suspected urologic injury. Semin Urol 1995;13: 9–24.

[16] Venn SN, Greenwell TJ, Mundy AR. Pelvic fracture injuries of the female urethra. BJU Int 1999;83: 626–30.

[17] Young JWR, Burgess AR. Radiological management of pelvic ring fractures. Baltimore (MD): Urban & Schwarzenberg; 1987. p. 22.

[18] Molligan HJ. Pelvic ring disruptions. In: McAninch JW, Jordan GH, Carroll PR, editors. Traumatic and reconstructive urology. Philadelphia: W.B. Saunders; 1996. p. 359.

[19] Pennal GF, Tile M, Waddell JP, et al. Pelvic disruption: assessment and classification. Clin Orth Res 1980;151:12.

[20] Koraitim MM. Pelvic fracture urethral injuries: the unresolved controversy. J Urol 1999;161:1433–41.

[21] Ziran BH, Chamberlin E, Shuler FD, et al. Delays and difficulties in the diagnosis of lower urologic injuries in the context of pelvic fractures. J Trauma 2005;58:533–7.

[22] Devine PC, Devine CJ. Posterior urethral injuries associated with pelvic fractures. Urology 1982;20: 467.

[23] Iselin CE, Webster GD. The significance of the open bladder neck associated with pelvic fracture urethral disruption defects. J Urol 1999;162:347–51.

[24] Pokorny M, Pontes JE, Pierce JM. Urological injuries associated with pelvic trauma. J Urol 1979;121: 455–7.

[25] Mundy AR. The role of delayed primary repair in the acute management of pelvic fracture injuries of the urethra. J Urol 1991;68:273–6.

[26] Andrich DE, Mundy AR. The nature of urethral injury in cases of pelvic fracture urethral trauma. J Urol 2001;165:1492–5.

[27] Mouraviev VB, Santucci RA. Cadaveric anatomy of pelvic fracture urethral distraction injury: most injuries are distal to the external urinary sphincter. J Urol 2005;173:869–72.

[28] Lim PHC, Chung HC. Initial management of acute urethral injuries. Br J Urol 1989;64:165–8.

[29] Colapinto V, McCallum RW. Injury to the male posterior urethra in the fractured pelvis: a new classification. J Urol 1977;118:575–80.

[30] Chapple C, Barbagli G, Jordan GH, et al. Consensus statement on urethral trauma. BJU Int 2004;93: 1195–202.

[31] Kotkin L, Koch MO. Impotence and incontinence after immediate realignment of posterior urethral trauma: result of injury or management? J Urol 1996;155:1600–3.

[32] Klosterman PW, McAninch JW. Urethral injuries. AUA update series vol. 8. Lesson 1989;32:249–56.

[33] Elliott DS, Barrett DM. Long term follow up and evaluation of primary realignment of posterior urethral disruptions. J Urol 1997;157:814.

[34] Morehouse DD, Belitsky P, MacKinnon K. Rupture of the posterior urethra. J Urol 1972;107:255–8.

[35] Webster GD, Guralnick ML. Reconstruction of posterior urethral disruption. Urol Clin N Am 2002;29:429–41.

[36] Dixon CM. Diagnosis and acute management of posterior urethral disruptions. In: McAninch JW, Jordan GH, Carroll PR, editors. Traumatic and reconstructive urology. Philadelphia: W.B. Saunders; 1996. p. 347–55.

[37] Kane NM, Francis IR, Ellis JH. The value of CT in the detection of bladder and posterior urethral injuries. AJR 1989;153:1243–6.

[38] Ali M, Safriel Y, Sclafani S, et al. CT signs of urethral injury. Radiographics 2003;23:951–66.

[39] Dixon C, Hricak H, McAninch JW. Magnetic resonance imaging of traumatic posterior urethral defects in pelvic crush injuries. J Urol 1992;148:1162–5.

[40] Goldman SM, Sandler CM, Corriere JN, et al. Blunt urethral trauma: a unified, anatomical mechanical classification. J Urol 1997;157:85–9.

[41] Sandler CM, Harris JH, Corriere JN, et al. Posterior urethral injuries after pelvic fracture. AJR 1981;137: 1233.

[42] Al Rifaei M, Eid NI, Al Rifaei A. Urethral injury secondary to pelvic fracture: anatomical and

functional classification. Scand J Urol Nephrol 2001;35:205–11.

[43] Richter ER, Morey AF. Urethral trauma. In: Wessells HB, McAninch JW, editors. Urological emergencies. Totowa (NJ): Humana Press; 2005. p. 57–69.

[44] Armenakas NA, McAninch JW. Acute anterior urethral injuries: diagnosis and initial management. In: McAninch JW, Jordan GH, Carroll PR, editors. Traumatic and reconstructive urology. Philadelphia: W.B. Saunders; 1996. p. 543–50.

[45] Hernandez J, Morey AF. Anterior urethral injury. World J Urol 1999;17:96–100.

[46] Park S, McAninch JW. Straddle injuries to the bulbar urethra: management and outcomes in 78 patients. J Urol 2004;171:722–5.

[47] Rosenstein DI, Morey AF, McAninch JW. Penile trauma. In: Graham SD, Glenn JF, editors. Glenn's urologic surgery. 5th edition. Philadelphia: Lippincott-Raven Publishers; 1998.

[48] Hall SJ, Wagner JR, Edelstein RA, et al. Management of gunshot injuries to the penis and anterior urethra. J Trauma 1995;38:439.

[49] Gomez RG, Castanheira AC, McAninch JW. Gunshot wounds to the male external genitalia. J Urol 1993;150:1147.

[50] Aliabadi H, Cass AS, Gleich P, et al. Self-inflicted foreign bodies involving the lower urinary tract and male genitals. Urology 1985;26:12–6.

[51] Rahman NU, Elliott SP, McAninch JW. Self-inflicted male urethral foreign body insertion. Endoscopic management and complications. BJU Int 2004;94:1051–3.

[52] Gottenger EE, Wagner JR. Penile fracture with complete urethral distruption. J Trauma 2000;49: 339–41.

[53] Witherington R, McKinney JE. An unusual case of anterior urethral injury. J Urol 1983;130:564.

[54] Vaidyanathan S, Soni BM, Dundas S, et al. Urethral cytology in spinal cord injury patients performing intermittent catheterization. Paraplegia 1994;32: 493–500.

[55] Barbagli G, Azzaro F, Menchi I, et al. Bacteriologic, histologic and ultrasonographic findings in strictures recurring after urethrotomy. Scand J Urol Nephrol 1995;29:193–5.

[56] Jordan GH. Urolume endoprosthesis for the treatment of recurrent bulbous urethral stricture. AUA Update Series 2000;19(3):18–23.

[57] Buchholz NP, Riehmann M, Gasser TC. Absence of urethral strictures with suprapubic urinary drainage during extracorporeal circulation. J Urol 1993;150: 337–9.

[58] Abdel-Hakim A, Bernstein J, Teijeira J, et al. Urethral stricture after cardiovascular surgery, a retrospective and prospective study. J Urol 1983;130: 1100.

[59] Bamshad BR, Poon MW, Stewart SC. Effect of cardiopulmonary bypass on urethral blood flow as measured by laser Doppler flowmetry. J Urol 1998;160: 2030–2.

[60] Baktavatsalam R. Complications relating to the urinary tract associated with bladder drained pancreatic transplantation. Br J Urol 1998;81(2): 219–23.

[61] Dumas MD, Bude RO, Sonda PL, et al. Urethral disruption with urinary extravasation: a delayed complication of pancreatic transplantation. Radiology 1996;201:761–5.

[62] Santucci RA, McAninch JW. Urethral reconstruction of strictures resulting from treatment of benign prostatic hypertrophy and prostate cancer. Urol Clin N Am 2002;29:417–27.

[63] Borboroglu PG, Sands JP, Roberts JL. Risk factors for vesicourethral anastomotic stricture after radical prostatectomy. Urology 2000;56:96–100.

[64] McConnell JD, Barry MJ, Bruskewitz RC. Benign prostatic hyperplasia: diagnosis and treatment. Clinical practice guidelines quick refernce guide. Rockville (MD): Agency for Health Care Policy and Research; 1994. p. 1–17.

[65] Zheng W, Vilos G, McCulloch S, et al. Electrical burn of urethra as a cause of stricture after transurethral resection. J Endourol 2000;14(2): 225–8.

[66] Sall M, Bruskewitz RC. Prostatic urethral strictures after transurethral microwave thermal therapy for benign prostatic hyperplasia. Urology 1997;50: 983–5.

[67] Orkin LA. Trauma to the bladder ureter and kidney. In: Sciarra JJ, editor. Gynecology and obstetrics. Philadelphia: JB Lippincott Co; 1991. p. 1–8.

[68] McAninch JW. Urethral injuries in female subjects following pelvic fractures. (Editorial comment). J Urol 1992;147:144.

[69] Perry MO, Hussmann DA. Urethral injuries in female subjects following pelvic fractures. J Urol 1992;147:139–43.

ELSEVIER
SAUNDERS

Urol Clin N Am 33 (2006) 87–95

UROLOGIC
CLINICS
of North America

Initial Management of Anterior and Posterior Urethral Injuries

Steven Brandes, MD

Division of Urologic Surgery, Washington University School of Medicine, Box 8242,
4960 Children's Place, St. Louis, MO 63110, USA

Précis

The key to the initial management of a urethral injury is prompt diagnosis, accurate staging of the injury, and properly selecting an intervention that minimizes the overall chances for the debilitating complications of incontinence, impotence, and urethral stricture. Although somewhat controversial, blunt traumatic posterior injuries generally are managed best by primary realignment (when feasible), straddle injuries of the bulbar urethra by suprapubic urinary diversion, and penetrating urethral injuries by primary repair and urinary diversion.

Urethral injuries are uncommon. Most are caused by blunt trauma from a pelvic fracture or straddle injury. Penetrating injuries are rare and usually are caused by a gunshot wound to the anterior urethra. Urethral injuries from pelvic fracture typically are associated with multiple other organ injuries (bladder, spleen, liver, and bowel). From such associated injuries, mortality rates can be as high as 30%. Initial management of the injured urethra is dependent on the degree and location of the injury, and the patient's hemodynamic stability and the associated injuries [1].

Posterior urethral injuries

Mechanism of blunt traumatic injuries

Classically, posterior urethral injuries are believed to be caused by shearing forces at fixation points. Recent studies, however, have questioned this mechanism of injury. The posterior urethra is believed to be fixed in place at two locations, at the membranous urethra, to the ischiopubic rami by the urogenital diaphragm, and at the prostatic urethra, to the symphysis by the puboprostatic ligaments. Urethral injuries traditionally are believed to be the result of major shearing forces at the prostatomembranous junction where the prostate is avulsed from a fixed urogenital diaphragm. With displacement of the prostate, the membranous urethra is stretched quickly and severely. When the puboprostatic ligaments also are ruptured, the highly elastic urethra can be stretched to considerable length without loss of continuity [2]. With complete avulsion ("prostatomembranous disruption"), the prostate is commonly displaced cephalad and the external urethral striated sphincter can be damaged [3,4]. In severe disruptions, the urogenital diaphragm laceration can extend into the bulbar urethra. With prostate disruption, the dorsal venous complex/Santorini's venous plexus is lacerated, resulting in massive pelvic hematoma. The pelvic hematoma frequently displaces the prostate further in a cephalad and posterior direction [5]. Other potential mechanisms of injury are shearing forces between a fixed prostate and a mobile bladder, resulting in bladder neck (BN) injury and, to a much lesser degree, direct laceration by pelvic bone fragments (rare) or urethral distraction/compression between the symphysis and pubic rami.

In contrast, mounting evidence shows that urethral disruption may not be at the prostatomembranous junction but rather a "bulbomembranous junction avulsion" [6–8]. In recent cadaveric studies, the perineal membrane was found to limit the undersurface of the urogenital

E-mail address: brandess@msnotes.wustl.edu

diaphragm, but no distinct superior membrane separated it from the prostate. The prostate, membranous urethra, and urethral sphincter are, therefore, believed to be one anatomical unit. During pelvic fracture, displacement of this anatomical unit and, thus, stretching of the membranous urethra is facilitated by disruption of the puboprostatic ligaments. As the membranous urethra is displaced, the bulbar urethra is fixed at the intact perineal membrane. This bulbo-membranous junction is believed to be weak and vulnerable to injury. In more severe cases, the perineal membrane also is disrupted and the bulbar urethra retracts into the perineum. Furthermore, after urethroplasty surgery for posterior urethral injuries, most (up to 85%) have some degree of extrinsic urethral sphincter function preserved [7].

Children

Injuries to the BN and prostatic urethra usually occur only in children with pelvic trauma [9,10]. The mechanism of injury is controversial. It is unclear whether the shearing forces between a fixed prostate and a mobile bladder result in BN injury or that the prepubertal and adolescent prostate is so small that the membranous urethral laceration extends transprostatic and into the BN [9,11].

Female urethra

Associated urethral injury in women with pelvic fractures is rare (<1% of pelvic fractures) because of the urethral short length, mobility, and lack of attachments to the pubic symphysis [12,13]. When urethral injury does occur, it is commonly a partial, anterior, and longitudinal laceration [14,15]. In extreme and rare cases, varying degrees of complete avulsion, associated vaginal lacerations, and pelvic fractures have occurred. Avulsion is predominantly at the proximal urethra, with occasional extension into the BN, and often associated with vaginal laceration [14]. Female urethral and BN injuries typically are not caused by shearing forces, as in the male urethra, but by direct laceration from sharp edges of fracture fragments. Concomitantly, injury to the vaginal vault also can occur from bony fragments and, thus, vaginal examination is important for all women with a pelvic fracture [14].

Grading of urethral injuries

To determine initial management, properly and accurately staging each urethral injury is

essential. The classic technique to diagnosing and grading an acute urethral injury is by retrograde urethrography. See the article elsewhere in this issue for details on this radiographic technique. Two urethral injury scales commonly are employed, the American Association for the Surgery of Trauma (AAST) [16] and Colapinto and McCallum [17] (later revised by Goldman S and colleagues [18]). AAST emphasizes degree of disruption (partial versus complete) and degree of urethral separation. Colapinto and McCallum emphasize fascial anatomy and the location of the urethral injury in relation to the urogenital diaphragm. See the article elsewhere in this issue for details on the grading schema.

Bedside flexible cystoscopy recently has been reported for diagnosing and managing a urethral injury. Kielb and colleagues [19] noted contusion—partial and complete disruption—could be diagnosed visually with reliable results. Major advantages to retrograde cystoscopy were that it seemed reliable and diagnostic, could be easily and quickly performed, could be performed in the supine position, and facilitated early catheterization in the emergency room with visual guidance (in 8 of 10 attempts) [19]. Although intriguing, major limitations of this series are that it has a small study cohort (10 patients), and follow-up is poor (6 out of 10 patients) and short (18 months).

Signs and symptoms

To decide on initial management of the injured urethra, a prompt diagnosis needs to be made. The diagnostic triad of blunt urethral injury is pelvic fracture, blood at the urethral meatus, and inability to void (or distended bladder). Ability to void, however, does not rule out the presence of a partial urethral injury. A voiding trial is discouraged, however, because massive urinary extravasation can occur and increase chances for pelvic and soft tissue fibrosis or infection. Overall, blood at the meatus is the most important sign of urethral injury— 98% and 75% sensitive for posterior and anterior urethral injuries, respectively [20]. Blood is expelled per meatus as a result of spasm of the bulbospongiosus muscle and often is apparent an hour after injury [21]. The amount of urethral bleeding correlates little with the severity of injury. Blood at the meatus should preclude attempts at catheterization until the urethra is imaged adequately. Other reliable signs of urethral injury are gross hematuria, scrotal, perineal, or penile ecchymosis or hematoma, difficulty passing a Foley, distended bladder, inability to void, or a "high riding" or "nonpalpable" prostate [22]. The sign of a "high riding prostate," however, is usually unreliable, as a result of examiner inexperience or the presence of a tense pelvic hematoma, which can blur the tissue planes and make palpation difficult (particularly in young men with small prostates). Female urethral injury is suspect when a pelvic fracture presents with vaginal bleeding or laceration (80%), urethrrhagia, hematuria, labial swelling, or inability to void [14].

Management

When one is deciding on the management of a posterior urethral injury, the method chosen should minimize the chances for the debilitating complications of incontinence, impotence, and urethral stricture, and avoid opening or infecting the pelvic hematoma. The ideal method of management, however, remains controversial. The age-old question on the etiology of posterior urethral injuries is whether the subsequent sequela from urethral injury is the result primarily of the injury itself or the result of, or worsened by, the method chosen for management? When the reports using open primary urethral repair and "rail-roading" techniques of yesteryear are excluded, contemporary series on posterior urethral injury give clear support that the etiology of urethral injury complications are a result of the injury itself [23]. Timing of the intervention typically is classified as "immediate" treatment when it takes place less than 48 hours after injury, "delayed primary" treatment after 2 to 14 days, and "deferred" treatment 3 months or more after injury.

Unless otherwise contraindicated, a Foley catheter is inserted during resuscitation to relieve urinary retention, to decompress the bladder before abdominal exploration, and to monitor urine output as an indicator of adequate resuscitation. When a urethral injury is suspected, catheterization is discouraged to prevent the potential conversion of a partial into a complete urethral injury (the potential for this occurring, however, is rare) [2]. A remote and theoretical potential exists in regards to infecting the pelvic hematoma [1]. Nonetheless, little evidence exists demonstrating that this risk for conversion occurs in practice, and, thus, one gentle attempt to place a Foley catheter in a partial disruption is reasonable [23]. Any resistance demands a retrograde urethrogram. In the young, conscious patient,

inability to pass a catheter usually is a result of sphincter spasm (a "tight" external sphincter) rather then a urethral injury. Furthermore, no convincing data exists demonstrating that a single, gentle catheterization attempt produces higher rates of infection or urethral stricture [23,24].

When a patient is referred with a urethral catheter already in place, and also has reported signs of urethral injury or a significant pelvic fracture, a high index of suspicion should be present for urethral injury. A pericatheter urethrogram should be performed before Foley removal. If extravasation is noted, the Foley catheter is kept in place, typically for 4 to 6 weeks, before re-imaging (Fig. 1).

Immediate surgical repair

Primary suturing of the severed urethral ends, although once commonly performed, has been abandoned because of high rates of postoperative impotence and incontinence, at 56% and 21%, respectively, in a literature meta-analysis [6]. Compared with a deferred treatment approach, stricture is less common at 49%, but impotence and incontinence are three times and five times worse, respectively. Other problems with primary suturing were potential release of the pelvic hematoma tamponade (risking uncontrolled bleeding), excessive urethral debridement and subsequent stricture (technically demanding), and the possibility of converting an incomplete to complete urethral injury during dissection [26]. Urethral catheter traction was also once a common

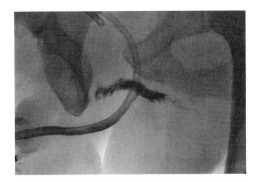

Fig. 1. 45 year-old with a urethral disruption injury after a motor cycle accident and pelvis ring disruption. Initially managed with endoscopic urethral realignment, a pericatheter urethrography is performed after 6 weeks. Note the persistent leak at the membranous urethra. The patient eventually failed his trial of primary realignment and underwent a successful deferred posterior urethroplasty.

practice, but it was associated with high complica-tion rates, thought to be caused by tissue ischemia of the sphincter and BN or to the prostate being pulled into an abnormal position when the uro-genital diaphragm was injured also [25,26]. Vest sutures were applied also for urethral realignment. This practice, however, also was abandoned as a result of the potential for prostate malrotation and misalignment [26].

Deferred treatment

After the abandonment of immediate primary repair in the 1970s, for the next two to three decades suprapubic urinary diversion followed by delayed primary repair has been the accepted general standard of care. This rings particularly true for the urologist who sees posterior urethral injuries only occasionally. By avoiding early in-tervention, iatrogenic injury is prevented and the injured soft-tissue is given time to heal.

In the acute trauma setting, when the urethra is injured and the bladder is distended, the supra-pubic (SP) tube usually can be placed percutane-ously, typically by Seldinger technique. Clear urine on SP tube placement suggests no major bladder injury. When gross hematuria is present a cystogram should be performed. When the bladder is empty (from recent micturition or concomitant bladder or BN injury), the SP tube is placed by open cystotomy. In this instance, care should be taken to avoid the prevesical/retropubic fascial planes so as not disrupt the pelvic hema-toma. Typically, the bladder is entered at the cephalad aspect of the dome. The bladder is ex-plored for concomitant bladder injuries. These ex-traperitoneal injuries are closed with absorbable suture from within the bladder. Prevesical drains typically are not used because they may increase the potential for pelvic hematoma infection. Over the next 3 to 6 months, the hematoma slowly reabsorbs and the prostate descends into a more normal position, and the scar tissue at the urethral disruption site becomes stable and mature. For complete urethral disruptions, this approach as-sumes an inevitable urethral stricture and need for delayed open urethroplasty or urethrotomy. The major advantage to deferred treatment is that in exchange for a high posterior urethral stricture rate is a low reported incidence of long-term impotence or incontinence. In a meta-analy-sis by Koritim [6], the overall complication rates for deferred treatment of posterior urethral inju-ries are posterior urethral stricture (97%), impo-tence (19%), and incontinence (4%) [6]. These

values of impotence and incontinence can be used as the goal standard for which all other inter-ventions are compared.

Primary realignment

Primary realignment by minimally invasive methods has become a common contemporary management option, particularly at high-volume trauma centers. Primary realignment of yesteryear was the reestablishment of urethral continuity by cumbersome "railroading" techniques, such as sound to sound (Davis interlocking sounds), retrograde sound to finger in BN, retrograde catheter placement under direct vision, or com-bined antegrade catheter sutured to retrograde catheter [26–29]. These techniques generally have been abandoned. Contemporary urethral realign-ment employs actual realignment by endoscopic guidance of flexible cystoscopes. Some have used a single flexible cystoscope and wire [30], whereas others employed two cystoscopes, one from above (antegrade) and one from below (retrograde), that keep the urethral ends in the same cephalad-cau-dal axis, followed by catheter placement across the disruption by Seldinger technique [27,29]. Sometimes the cystoscope from above can be passed antegrade through the BN, across the dis-rupted membranous-bulb, and into the disrupted distal urethral edge. If this fails, a second surgeon cystoscopes from below, the light source to the an-tegrade scope turned off, and the antegrade scope advanced toward the light. If this fails, realign-ment is performed under combined endoscopic and biplanar fluoroscopic guidance (Fig. 2). A ra-dio-opaque guide wire under visual and fluoro-scopic control is also commonly used to help bridge the urethral avulsion gap (Fig. 3) [31]. The urethral catheter usually is maintained for 4 to 6 weeks and acts as a guide that allows the distracted urethral ends to come together, in the same plane, as the pelvic hematoma slowly reabsorbs. These minimally invasive techniques can be performed immediately or in a delayed fashion.

Some worry that endoscopic attempts at re-alignment may induce or predispose the pelvic hematoma to infection as a result of irrigation during cystoscopy. Such iatrogenic pelvic infec-tion has never been reported. Nonetheless, these concerns are theoretical and clearly do not out-weigh the real benefits of primary realignment.

Immediate primary realignment

Immediate primary approach usually is per-formed in the stable trauma patient with a short urethral disruption distance. Associated injuries

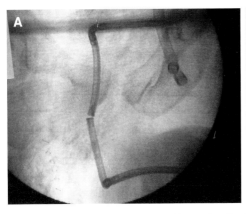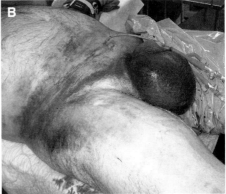

Fig. 2. (*A*) Type 3 urethral avulsion injury with associated pelvic fracture. Note endoscopic and fluoroscopic delayed (3 days post injury) primary realignment with the use of two flexible cystoscopes, one retrograde and the other antegrade through a suprapubic tube tract. (*B*) Same patient after primary realignment. Note the suprapubic tube, the massively distended scrotum from blood and urine extravasation, and the right lower quadrant ecchymoses.

to the BN, bladder, or rectum demand immediate exploration but not necessarily immediate urethral realignment. Present series on immediate primary realignment are generally small and with short follow-up, but when compared with urinary diversion alone, rates are comparable for incontinence (1% versus 4%) and impotence (28% versus 19%) [32,33]. For all primary realignment cases (early and delayed) the stricture rates are decreased, (53% versus 97%) [6]. In the only long-term follow-up study on immediate primary realignment, Elliot and Barrett [28] demonstrated

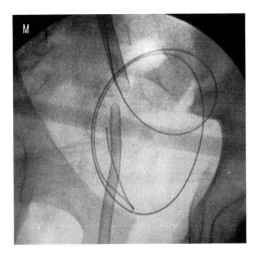

Fig. 3. After failed attempts at endoscopic realignment, a floppy-tipped guide wire is passed antegrade into the prevesical and periprostatic space to facilitate primary realignment of a posterior urethral disruption injury.

with 53 patients and a 10.5 year follow-up, that rates of impotence, stress incontinence, and strictures, are 21%, 3.7%, and 68%, respectively. These complication rates are low and nicely compare with Koritim's meta-analysis [6]. Demonstrable lower stricture rates to deferred treatment were demonstrated also.

Delayed primary realignment

In the unstable or multisystem trauma patient, realignment often is delayed a few days to weeks (typically 2 to 14 days). Here, the patient is first managed by damage control and resuscitated in the intensive care unit while the urine is diverted by SP tube placement. Once the patient is stable, warm, and the acidosis and coagulopathy corrected, delayed urethral realignment is performed. This procedure can be combined conveniently with early open reduction and internal fixation of the associated unstable pelvic fractures [34]. SP tubes commonly are discouraged by orthopedists because they often feel the tubes can compromise anterior exposure for internal fixation of the pelvis. This type of interference with the ilial-inguinal incision generally can be avoided by placing the SP tube high, at least 2 to 3 cm cephalad to the pubic bone. SP tubes also are purported in orthopedic circles to increase the rate for hardware infection; however, no literature exists that supports such assertions [34]. Another advantage to early realignment is that the SP tube placed at the time of initial injury usually can be removed. Furthermore, in a delayed approach, the patient is stable and can tolerate a potentially time-consuming realignment procedure. In general, primary realignment takes up to 1.25 hours (mean) [29,34].

An ingenious method at delayed primary realignment of complete urethral avulsion was the use of magnetic tipped catheters to facilitate stenting the urethra [35]. Although reported to be effective (85% stented) and safe, with acceptably low and comparably efficacious complication rates (50% stricture rate, 14% impotence), its limited volume of use did not warrant continued production. Such catheters are not available now commercially.

Endourologic and radiologic techniques for realignment, theoretically, should not affect potency or urinary continence because no manipulation occurs of the periprostatic tissues or neurovascular bundles. Most contemporary series on delayed primary realignment are small, but when compared with urinary diversion alone, rates are comparable for incontinence (4% versus 4%) and impotence (23% versus 19%), whereas rates of stricture formation for early and delayed series are decreased (53% versus 97%) [6,23]. In the long-term follow-up study of 8.8 years in 96 patients by Mouraviev and colleagues [36], delayed early primary realignment (57 patients) provided better outcomes and fewer complications then deferred repair (39 patients) for all parameters. These results included stricture rates (49% versus 100%), impotence (33.6% versus 42.1%), and incontinence (17.7% versus 24.9%), and further support the concept that impotence and incontinence after urethral disruption are the result of the injury itself not the immediate treatment method.

Aside from aligning the prostate and urethra, eventual stricture lengths also may be decreased with primary realignment and so make later urethral reconstruction easier [10]. Short urethral strictures can be managed more easily and are more amenable potentially to urethrotomy or dilation (in up to one half of cases) [37]. Urethrotomy success, however, was not durable (<40% at 3 years); therefore, the goal to managing urethral disruption often is not to prevent urethral stricture formation but to minimize the length and peri-urethral fibrosis of the strictures that do occur and so ease subsequent treatments [38].

Bladder neck

With pelvic disruption, injury to the BN can occur, although rare. Early repair of a BN injury avoids incontinence, infection, and fistula formation, it is believed. Diagnosis of the injury can be made by cystogram or by palpation at the time of bladder exploration. For simple lacerations, effective management is typically urinary drainage by prolonged catheter drainage. For complete disruption/avulsion, repair often is recommended. Typically, this repair is technically demanding, and in the unstable patient, repair often is better delayed. To minimize potential scarring and BN entrapment, Turner-Warwick [3,25] also advocated omental pedicle flap mobilization and BN coverage. Furthermore, male children typically are more susceptible than adults to BN injury and thus post-traumatic incontinence [9,11]. In women, injuries to the BN are caused by shearing forces of bony fragments through the urethra and vaginal vault. Associated vaginal lacerations are common, as is an increased incidence of vesicovaginal fistula.

Female urethra

In female urethral injuries, urethrography can demonstrate extravasation of contrast from areas of laceration. Others feel that the acutely traumatized female urethra is best assessed for injury by urethroscopy [39]. In sharp contrast to the management of male urethral injuries, women with pelvic fractures and proximal urethral disruptions are recommended to undergo immediate retropubic exploration with realignment of the urethral ends or primary anastomosis over a catheter [14,40]. When these injuries are managed by only proximal urinary diversion, urethrovaginal fistulas or obliterative urethral strictures commonly occur [40]. To further prevent fistula formation, concomitant vaginal lacerations also need repair at that time (transvaginally). For lacerations of the distal urethra, the continence mechanism is not at risk and thus the urethra can be managed by catheterization (or proximal urethral advancement) and primary closure of the vaginal laceration [12,13]. Unfortunately, diagnosis of female urethral injury often is missed initially and present in a delayed fashion with obstructive voiding, urinary retention, or urinary incontinence (vesicovaginal or urethrovaginal fistula).

Anterior urethral injuries

In contrast to traumatic posterior urethral injuries, anterior urethral injuries typically are caused by direct injury to the penis and urethra, have few associated injuries, and low morbidity. Classically, anterior urethral injuries result from a "straddle" injury or a kick or blow to the perineum, wherein the bulbar urethra is crushed against the pubic bone. Penetrating urethral injuries (gunshots or stab wounds) also can involve the anterior urethra. Other causes for anterior urethral injury are severe penile fracture, iatrogenic trauma from catheterization, or insertion of foreign bodies. Signs of urethral injury from a straddle injury usually are apparent by high index of suspicion (by mechanism), blood at the meatus (the most important predictor), tender or ecchymotic perineum, and the classic "purple butterfly" sign [1].

Management

The initial management of all urethral injuries is resuscitation of the patient and the diagnosis of all potentially life-threatening injuries. The key to managing an anterior urethral injury is making a prompt diagnosis. Missed injuries can result in infection of the extravasated urine and blood, with possible development of an abscess or necrotizing fasciitis of the scrotum and perineum.

1. Contusion

Contusion of the urethra is a mucosal injury that heals without significant scarring. Such injuries typically occur when a Foley with an inflated balloon is removed traumatically or the balloon is accidentally inflated in the anterior urethra. On cystoscopy, the urethelial lining is inflamed, but no urethral laceration is present. Management is expectant, and no catheterization is required [1].

2. Lacerations

Lacerations of the urethra result in extravasation of urine and blood from the urethra that spreads along the fascial planes of the perineum and penis. If Buck's fascia is intact, extravasation is confined to the penis, giving a "sleeve-like" penile ecchymosis and swelling. When Buck's fascia is injured, extravasation extends into the perineum, as limited by Colle's fascia, and so creates the classical "butterfly sign" hematoma. The ecchymoses can also extend on to the anterior abdominal wall, along Scarpa's fascia [1].

Partial laceration. Management of partial urethral lacerations typically entails suprapubic urinary diversion or primary realignment/urethral catheterization for 1 to 2 weeks. Attempts at "blind" catheterization can risk converting an incomplete into a complete urethral tear. Incomplete lacerations usually heal rapidly and with

a low stricture rate. Before catheter removal an urethrogram is obtained to confirm urethral healing. When strictures do occur they are typically short or flimsy and can be managed effectively by urethrotomy [1].

Complete laceration/straddle injury. In a delayed fashion, these injuries typically result in proximal bulbar urethral strictures, (mean length = 1.8 cm) [41]. Extrapolating from the experience with posterior urethral avulsion injuries, intuitively, early endoscopic realignment over a Foley catheter for the anterior urethral injury should produce fewer strictures then just SP tube placement. The data, however, are somewhat contradictory. The San Francisco General group recently reported its experience with 78 straddle injuries to the bulbar urethra [41]. Contrary to popular convention, the primary realignment group more commonly required urethroplasty (17% versus 9%) and, moreover, complex flap or graft urethroplasty over suprapubic urinary diversion alone. The explanations for this are unclear. Of the strictures, 92% eventually required an excision and primary anastomotic urethroplasty, with a 95% success rate at 25 months [41].

When Buck's fascia is disrupted, urine can extend into the scrotum and abdominal wall. Extensive extravasation requires close observation as infection, tissue necrosis, or fasciitis may present in a delayed fashion. Aside from urinary

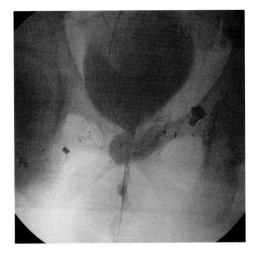

Fig. 4. Gunshot wound to the prostatic urethra. Note contrast extravasation from the prostatic urethra and primary realignment with endoscopic and fluoroscopic retrograde placement of a guide wire and subsequent Council-type Foley catheter.

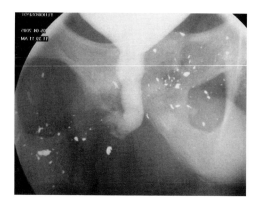

Fig. 5. Gunshot wound to the membranous and proximal bulbar urethra. Note the loss of the right inferior pubic ramus. Multiple other intra-abdominal injuries made the patient unstable and thus the urethral injury was managed in a damage control fashion by percutaneous suprapubic tube placement. Deferred management eventually required a posterior urethroplasty and inferior pubectomy.

diversion, these complications may require tissue debridement of devitalized tissue, subcutaneous drainage, or intravenous antibiotics. Although debridement should be aggressive, corpus spongiosum debridement should be minimized because the ecchymotic and visibly contused spongoisum often is not necrotic. Preservation of urethral tissue should be maximized so as to facilitate subsequent reconstruction [1].

Penetrating anterior urethral injuries

Gunshot wounds (GSWs) to the urethra are uncommon and occur in up to 6.5% of all civilian urologic GSWs [42,43]. GSWs to the penis injure the pendulous or bulbar urethra in 18% to 57% [43–46]. Furthermore, of GSWs to the perineum, roughly half have an associated urethra injury [42]. Reliable signs for penetrating urethral injury are penetrating wounds to the penis or perineum, blood at the penile meatus, gross hematuria, or a high index of suspicion [42–45]. The amount of contrast extravasation on urethrography usually does not correlate with the severity of the injury (Fig. 4) [43].

For stab wounds and low velocity GSWs to the anterior urethra, a primary open repair typically is effective, durable, and, thus, preferred. Comparative studies of low velocity anterior urethral GSWs with partial urethral transections demonstrate stricture rates of up to 78% for urinary diversion or primary realignment, compared with

only 12% for primary urethral repair [46]. Surgical management entails urethral mobilization, conservative debridement, and primary tension-free anastomosis of spatulated urethral ends, over a Foley catheter. Because of a rich blood supply, when the corpora spongiosum is contused it can seem necrotic [43,47]. Visual assessment of corporal viability often is unreliable. Conservative urethral debridement is essential to avoid large defects that are difficult to reconstruct [43,47]. Penetrating posterior urethral injuries, however, are difficult to access and typically are managed by primary realignment or proximal urinary diversion and deferred reconstruction (Fig. 5).

For high-velocity GSWs or shot-gun blasts, extensive blast effect and urethral loss are typical. Long urethral defects cannot be re-approximated without tension, and risk high rates of stricture, fistula, and ventral penile curvature [11,43]. Extensive urethral injuries are best managed by a staged repair of urethral marsupialization and suprapubic urinary diversion [46,47]. At a planned second stage, three or more months later, a modified Thiersch-Duplay urethroplasty can be performed.

References

[1] Klosterman PW, McAninch JW. Urethral injuries. AUA update series 1989;8(32).
[2] Mitchell JP. Injuries to the urethra. Br J Urol 1968; 40:649.
[3] Turner-Warwick R. A personal view of the immediate management of pelvic fracture urethral injuries. Urol Clin North Am 1977;4:81.
[4] Pokorny M, Pontes JE, Pierce JM Jr. Urological injuries associated with pelvic trauma. J Urol 1979; 121:455.
[5] Clark SS, Prudencio RF. Lower urinary tract injuries associated with pelvic fractures: diagnosis and management. Surg Clin North Am 1972;52:183.
[6] Koraitim MM, Marzouk ME, Atta MA, et al. Risk factors and mechanisms of urethral injury in pelvic fractures. Br J Urol 1996;71:876.
[7] Andrich DE, Mundy AR. The nature of urethral injury in cases of pelvic fracture urethral trauma. J Urol 2001;165(5):1492.
[8] Mouraviev VB, Coburn M, Santucci RA. The treatment of posterior urethral disruption associated with pelvic fractures: comparative experience of early realignment versus delayed urethroplasty. J Urol 2005; 173(3):873.
[9] Snyder H, Williams DI. Urethral injuries in children. Br J Urol 1977;48:663.
[10] Devine CJ Jr, Jordan GH, Devine PC. Primary realignment of the disrupted prostatomembranous urethra. Urol Clin North Am 1989;16:291.

[11] Merchant WC, Gibbons MD, Gonzales ET. Trauma to the bladder neck, trigone, and vagina in children. J Urol 1984;131:747.

[12] Flaherty JJ, Kelly R, Burnett B, et al. Relationship of pelvic bone fracture patterns to injuries of urethra and bladder. J Urol 1968;99:297.

[13] Pokorny M, Pontes JE, Pierce JM Jr. Urologic injuries associated with pelvic trauma. J Urol 1979;121:455.

[14] Perry MO, Husmann DA. Urethral injuries in female subjects following pelvic fractures. J Urol 1992;147:139.

[15] Venn SN, Greenwell TJ, Mundy AR. Pelvic fracture injuries of the female urethra. BJU Int 1999;83:626.

[16] Moore EE, Cogbill TH, Malagoni MA, et al. Organ injury scaling. Surg Clin North Am 1995;75:293.

[17] Colapinto V, McCollum RW. Injury to the male posterior urethra in fractured pelvis: a new classification. J Urol 1977;118:575.

[18] Goldman SM, Sandler CM, Corriere JN Jr, et al. Blunt urethral trauma: a unified, anatomical mechanical classification. J Urol 1997;157:85.

[19] Kielb SJ, Voeltz ZL, Wolf JS. Evaluation and management of traumatic posterior urethral disruption with flexible cystourethroscopy. J Trauma 2001;50:36–40.

[20] McAninch JW. Traumatic injuries to the urethra. J Trauma 1981;21:291.

[21] Lowe MA, Mason JT, Luna GK, et al. Risk factors for urethral injuries in men with traumatic pelvic fractures. J Urol 1988;140:506.

[22] Spirnak JP. Pelvic fracture and injury to the lower urinary tract. Surg. Clin North Am 1988;68:1057.

[23] Kotkin L, Koch MO. Impotence and incontinence after immediate realignment of posterior urethral trauma: result of injury or management. J Urol 1996;155:1600.

[24] Coffield KS, Weems WL. Experience with management of posterior urethral injury associated with pelvic fracture. J Urol 1977;117:772.

[25] Turner-Warwick R. Prevention of complications resulting from pelvic fracture urethral injuries- and from their surgical management. Urol Clin North Am 1989;16:335.

[26] Webster GD, Mathes GL, Selli C. Prostatomembranous urethral injuries: a review of the literature and a rational approach to their management. J Urol 1983;130:898.

[27] Elliott DS, Barrett DM. Long-term follow-up and evaluation of primary realignment of posterior urethral disruptions. J Urol 1997;157:814.

[28] Deweerd JH. Immediate realignment of posterior urethral injury. Urol Clin North Am 1977;4:75.

[29] Follis HW, Koch MO, McDougal WS. Immediate management of prostatomembranous urethral disruptions. J Urol 1992;147:1259.

[30] Gheiler EL, Frontera R Jr. Immediate primary realignment of prostatomembranous urethral disruptions using endourologic techniques. Urology 1997;49(4):596.

[31] Gelbard MK, Heyman AM, Weintraub P. A technique for immediate realignment and catheterization of the disrupted prostatomembranous urethra. J Urol 1989;142:52.

[32] Koch MO, Kirchner FK. Endoscopic realignment of prostatomembranous urethral disruptions. Atlas Urol Clin North Am 1998;6(2):1–12.

[33] Londergan TA, Gundersen LH, Van Every MJ. Early fluoroscopic realignment for traumatic urethral injuries. Urology 1997;49:101.

[34] Moudouni SM, Patard JJ, Manunta A, et al. Early endoscopic realignment of post-traumatic posterior urethral disruption. Urology 2001;57:628–32.

[35] Porter JR, Takayama TK, Defalco AJ. Traumatic posterior urethral injury and early realignment using magnetic urethral catheters. J Urol 1997;158:425.

[36] Mouraviev VB, Santucci RA. Cadaveric anatomy of pelvic fracture urethral distraction injury: most injuries are distal to the external urinary sphincter. J Urol 2005;173(3):869.

[37] Ennemoser O, Colleselli K, Reissigl A, et al. Post-traumatic posterior urethral stricture repair: anatomy, surgical approach and long-term results. J Urol 1997;157(2):499.

[38] Mundy A. The role of delayed primary repair in the acute management of pelvic fracture injuries of the urethra. Br J Urol 1991;68:273.

[39] McAninch JW. Urethral injuries in female subjects following pelvic fractures (editorial comment). J Urol 1992;147:139.

[40] Morehouse DD. Management of posterior urethral rupture: a personal view. Br J Urol 1988;61:375.

[41] Park S, McAninch JW. Straddle injuries to the bulbar urethra: management and outcomes in 78 patients. J Urol 2004;(2, Pt 1):722.

[42] Archbold JAA, Barros D'Sa AAB, Morrison E. Genito-urinary tract injuries of civil hostilities. Br J Surg 1981;68:625.

[43] Brandes SB, Buckman RF, Chelsky MJ, et al. External genitalia gunshot wounds: a ten-year experience with fifty-six cases. J Trauma 1995;39:266.

[44] Miles BJ, Poffenberger RJ, Farah RN, et al. Management of penile gunshot wounds. Urology 1990;36:318.

[45] Gomez RG, Castanheria AC, McAninch JW. Gunshot wounds to the male external genitalia. J Urol 1993;150:1147.

[46] Hausmann DA, Boone TB, Wilson WT. Management of low velocity gunshot wounds to the anterior urethra: the role of primary repair versus urinary diversion alone. J Urol 1993;150:70.

[47] Selkowitz SM. Penetrating high velocity genitourinary injuries. Urology 1977;9:371.

ELSEVIER
SAUNDERS

Urol Clin N Am 33 (2006) 97–109

**UROLOGIC
CLINICS
of North America**

Reconstruction and Management of Posterior Urethral and Straddle Injuries of the Urethra

Gerald H. Jordan, MD, FACS, FAAP[a,b,*], Ramón Virasoro, MD[a],
Ehab A. Eltahawy, MD[a]

[a]Department of Urology, Eastern Virginia Medical School, 400 West Brambleton Avenue,
Suite 100, Norfolk, VA 23510, USA
[b]Devine Center for Genitourinary Reconstructive Surgery, Sentara Norfolk General Hospital,
400 West Brambleton Avenue, Suite 100, Norfolk, VA 23510, USA

Urethral stricture disease was formerly almost always associated with inflammatory conditions of the urethra. That usually meant gonococcal urethritis. However, trauma is also a frequent cause of urethral stricture. With the development of catheters and endoscopy, iatrogenic injuries to the urethra have increasingly been the cause of strictures. One common mechanism of trauma to the urethra is the fall-astride injury. Another very common injury to the urethra is the urethral distraction defect associated with pelvic fracture. Pelvic fracture urethral distraction defects occur with about 10% of pelvic fractures. The lesion usually affects the bulbomembranous junction, but can involve any portion of the membranous urethra. In the case of perineal straddle trauma, the injury usually involves the anterior urethra and, depending on the angle of the fall, can involve a section from the penoscrotal junction to the bulbomembranous junction. Today, fall-astride injury is probably the most common cause of anterior urethral stricture. Probably every instance of short-length narrow-caliber bulbous stricture is the result of straddle trauma, either recognized or unrecognized at the time of injury. Nowadays, inflammatory strictures are still seen, but they are most commonly associated with lichen sclerosus (balanitis xerotica obliterans) or catheter-induced urethritis. This article will deal only with those strictures associated with perineal straddle trauma or pelvic fracture urethral distraction defects.

Anatomy

To understand the issue of strictures associated with perineal straddle trauma or pelvic fracture urethral distraction defects, a thorough understanding of the urethral anatomy is essential. As a result of a World Health Organization Consensus Conference about trauma to the urinary tract, the urologic community has come to an agreement on classifying the six segments of the urethra (Fig. 1). This article discusses the bulbous urethra and the membranous urethra. The bulbous urethra has four distinguishing characteristics (Fig. 2): (1) It is eccentrically placed relative to the bulk of the corpus spongiosum; (2) it is located where the bulbous portion of the corpus spongiosum is invested by the midline fusion of the ischial cavernosus musculature; (3) It is located where the bulk of the corpus spongiosum is the greatest; and (4) its lumen is, in most patients, the largest portion of the anterior urethra.

Meanwhile, the membranous urethra is the only segment of the male urethra that is not surrounded by another structure. By comparison, the prostatic urethra is invested by the bulk of the prostate and the anterior urethra is invested by the spongy erectile tissue of the corpus spongiosum and the glans penis. The membranous urethra extends from the apex of the prostate to the bulbomembranous junction. Proximally, the membranous urethra contains the external smooth muscle sphincter as well as the external rhabdosphincter.

---

* Corresponding author.

E-mail address: ghjordan@sentara.com
(G.H. Jordan).

0094-0143/06/$ - see front matter © 2005 Elsevier Inc. All rights reserved.
doi:10.1016/j.ucl.2005.11.007

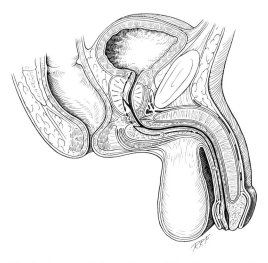

Fig. 1. Sections of the urethra as defined by the World Health Organization Consensus Conference. (*1*) Fossa navicularis. (*2*) Pendulous urethra. (*3*) Bulbous urethra. (*4*) Membranous urethra. (*5*) Prostatic urethra. (*6*) Bladder neck. (*Adapted from* Devine CJ Jr, Angermeier KW. Anatomy of the penis and male perineum. AUA Update Series 1994:8(2):11.)

The deep vasculature of the penis depends on the common penile artery, which is the extension of the deep internal pudendal artery, after the superficial blood supply has been given off. The venous drainage was well described by the dissections of Aboseif and Lue [1] and is not usually a factor in urethral reconstruction. Figs. 3 and 4 show the arterial and venous drainage of the penis.

Posterior urethral distraction defects

Physiopathology and location of injury

Distraction defects of the posterior urethra are always a result of trauma associated with pelvic fracture. Pokorny and colleagues [2] proposed four mechanisms of injury to the posterior urethra. These mechanisms correlate with the classification of types of distraction defects first proposed by Colapinto and McCallum [3]. That classification has been revised recently by Goldman and colleagues [4]. The most frequent mechanism is the diametric or Malgaigne's fracture. This type of fracture is the result of a force applied over the femur. The upward displacement of the symphysis pubis provokes the rupture of the puboprostatic ligament, and can stretch the membranous urethra to the point of rupture. The second mechanism postulated is the bilateral fracture of both superior and inferior pubic

rami, leading to a posteroinferior displacement of the ruptured bone fragment against the membranous urethra, thus perhaps causing the bone fragment to act as a guillotine. The third mechanism involves diastasis of the symphysis pubis with rupture of one puboprostatic ligament, thus tearing the perineal membrane from the opposite bone. The fourth mechanism speculates a direct injury to the posterior urethra by a spicule of the fractured pubis close to the midline. In those cases, the prostatic urethra and the bladder can also be injured. What is not addressed by either classification, is the vertical injury to the membranous urethra and prostatic urethra. In the authors' experience, this vertical injury to the membranous urethra and prostatic urethra is associated with injuries that cause wide diastasis of the pubis. Traditionally the location of the pelvic fracture urethral distraction has been described as being at the prostatomembranous junction. However, many articles in the literature suggest that the most frequent site of distraction is at the bulbomembranous junction (Fig. 5). This is also the opinion of the World Health Organization Consultation on urethral trauma in 2004 [5]. A recent study on 10 male cadavers, conducted by Mouraviev and Santucci [6], supports evidence that the bulbomembranous junction is the area most frequently injured in pelvic fracture urethral distraction defects.

In the past, conventional wisdom held that the external urethral sphincter was inevitably injured during these injuries. The current literature, however, suggests that the external sphincter mechanism, including both the rhabdosphincter as well as the external smooth muscle sphincter, can remain intact in many cases of pelvic fracture urethral distraction defects [7,8].

Even so, in young males, the injury can damage the prostatic urethra and, in females, the injury can harm the bladder neck. Traumatic injuries to the urethra can result in erectile dysfunction and urinary incontinence, and can be associated with abscess and fistula formation. This article, however, will deal only with the management of the distraction defect per se.

Acute presentation and diagnostic techniques

The classic findings of pelvic fracture associated urethral distraction are:

The patient has a pelvic fracture.
There is blood at the meatus.

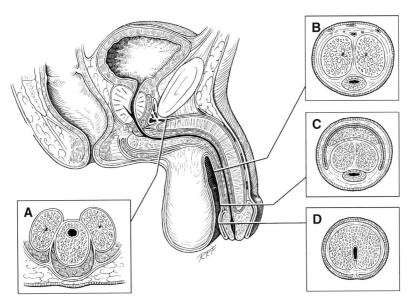

Fig. 2. Cross-sectional anatomy of the anterior urethra. In (*A*), the bulbous urethra is eccentrically placed with regards to the bulk of the bulbospongiosum. In (*B*) and (*C*), the urethra becomes more centrally placed, with the fossa navicularis (*D*) becoming ventrally displaced with regards to the bulk of the spongy erectile tissue of the corpus spongiosum. (*Main figure adapted from* Devine CJ Jr, Angermeier KW. Anatomy of the penis and male perineum. AUA Update Series. 1994:8(2):11. *A–D from* Jordan GH. Complications of interventional techniques of urethral stricture disease: direct visual internal urethrostomy, stents, and laser. In: Carson CC, editor. Topics in clinical urology complications of interventional techniques. New York: Igaku-Shoin; 1996. p. 86–94.)

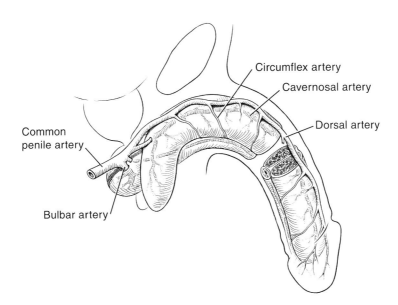

Fig. 3. Deep vasculature of the penis and urethra. (*From* Horton CE, Stecker JF, Jordan GH. Management of erectile dysfunction and genital reconstruction following trauma and transsexualism. In: McCarthy JG, May JW Jr, Littler JW, editors. Plastic surgery, volume 6. Philadelphia: WB Saunders; 1990. p. 4213–45.)

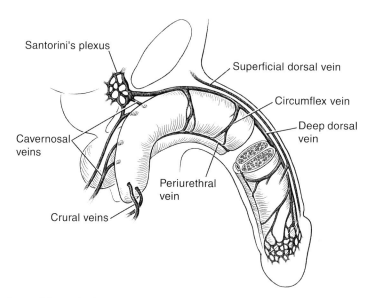

Fig. 4. Venous drainage of the penis. (*From* Horton CE, Stecker JF, Jordan GH. Management of erectile dysfunction and genital reconstruction following trauma and transsexualism. In: McCarthy JG, May JW Jr, Littler JW, editors. Plastic surgery, volume 6. Philadelphia: WB Saunders; 1990. p. 4213–45.)

On rectal examination the prostate appears to be high riding or difficult to palpate.
The patient has not been able to void.

However, these classic presenting signs or symptoms are not always present. Ziran and

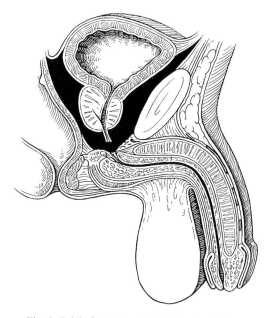

Fig. 5. Pelvic fracture urethral distraction injury.

colleagues found that 17% to 21% of lower urinary tract injuries associated with pelvic fracture can be initially missed [9]. Prompt identification of the injury is essential to reduce morbidity. The initial management may in many cases serve only to reduce subsequent morbidity. However, investigators have recently proposed that certain techniques of initial management can in fact not only reduce the disruption in the urethral continuity, but can also contribute therapeutically to healing.

The retrograde urethrogram is the cornerstone study for initial diagnosis. The retrograde urethrogram demonstrates whether or not the watertight continuity of the urethra is intact. Ideally, the patient should be placed in a lateral oblique position. However, in the case of pelvic fracture, this position can be very uncomfortable for the patient. The goal of the retrograde urethrogram is not strictly to identify the anatomy of the injury, but rather to demonstrate whether or not the continuity of the urethral lumen has been disrupted. In all pelvic fractures, a cystogram or direct examination of the bladder must also be performed to exclude concomitant bladder injury.

Some medical centers now use flexible urethroscopy to diagnose these injuries. Supporters of this approach say that it not only helps diagnose the injury, but it also can facilitate the placement of an aligning urethral catheter, and thereby can initiate active treatment of the distraction defect. However, not everyone agrees with this approach and the initial management of the injured posterior urethra remains somewhat controversial. Should the watertight continuity of the urethral lumen be interrupted as demonstrated by contrast extravasation, most experts recommend that blind catheter placement be avoided. In some cases, if a urologist is available at the time of patient presentation, an attempt at catheterization may be made. Careful retrograde flexible urethroscopy can also be done and is a safe diagnostic procedure. As mentioned, in some cases, an aligning catheter can then be placed through the distraction defect. Some defects can be total while in some cases only a partial portion of the circumference of the urethra is distracted. Placement of an aligning catheter, in the authors' opinion, should be viewed as an adjuvant to diversion with a suprapubic catheter. However, at some medical centers, physicians are comfortable with the practice of inserting the aligning Foley catheter as the only initial form of diversion.

Immediate management options available include suprapubic tube placement and delayed repair, first proposed by Johanson [10]; primary suture of the torn ends of the urethra, first described by Young [11]; and primary realignment of the two ends through open surgery [10] or endoscopically [12], without traction. Each procedure has its own advantages and disadvantages, as well as advocates and opponents.

At Sentara Norfolk General Hospital, the preferred procedure is to insert a 16 F suprapubic catheter via an open technique, and defer the urethral repair.

The authors place, when possible, an aligning catheter (eg, 14 F silicone) for approximately 6 to 8 weeks. The suprapubic catheter can be placed immediately at the dome of the bladder by extending a small incision into the peritoneal cavity, thus identifying the dome of the bladder. This technique allows the surgeon to place the catheter right at the dome of the bladder. Furthermore, with this technique, the surgeon can directly inspect the entire interior of the bladder and stay away from the pelvic hematoma. If the case involves pelvic internal fixation hardware, the technique also provides the surgeon access to the bladder without disturbing that hardware.

At the time of delayed reconstruction, suprapubic access to the bladder allows antegrade flexible cystourethroscopy in combination with retrograde urethrography. This combined technique provides excellent information regarding length of the distraction, and allows visualization of the bladder neck. However, accurate assessment of bladder neck function is not necessarily possible.

The appearance of the bladder neck on cystogram and on visualization does not absolutely predict continence [13]. The proper placing of the patient in a steep lateral oblique position is essential to accurately assess the length of distraction.

Definitive urethroplasty takes place at least 3 months after injury. In most cases, injuries are repaired after 6 months. This time frame allows the pelvic hematoma to reabsorb and settles down the true length of the urethral disruption, which is less than 2 cm in most cases. In practice, the delay between the time of injury and repair normally depends on factors other than reabsorption of the hematoma. These factors include associated orthopedic injuries and the potential for deep venous thromboses. Many patients with urethral disruption injuries now survive trauma that not long ago would have killed them.

Operative procedures

Most experts agree that a primary anastomotic technique is the best way to reconstruct these lesions. Many investigators report a success rate of 90% to 97%. The authors believe that the perineal approach is suitable for almost all posterior urethral disruption defects. The retropubic access, described by Waterhouse [14], is not used at Sentara Norfolk General Hospital. However, in some cases where there are concomitant injuries to the rectum and bladder neck, surgeons should consider a combined perineal and abdominal approach. Whether the surgeon completely excises the area of fibrosis or creates a posterior incision of the fibrosis, the goal is to allow a tension-free anastomosis of the anterior urethral lumen to the posterior urethral lumen. This aspect of the surgery is a matter of the surgeon's preference.

One-stage perineal anastomotic repair of the membranous urethra

Posterior urethral distractions are short in most cases. The goal is a tension-free, widely spatulated anastomosis, with optimal epithelial apposition.

Broad-spectrum intravenous antibiotics based on the results of the urine culture are initiated 24 hours prior to surgery. Before positioning the patient in the exaggerated lithotomy position, endoscopy is performed through the meatus and again through the suprapubic tube sinus. Endoscopy on the table is useful to identify concomitant vesicolithiasis and allows evaluation of the urethra proximal and distal to the distraction defect. Antegrade cystoscopy is performed with a rigid cystoscope under anesthesia. The cytoscope is gently manipulated. If the impulse of the instrument tip is easily felt on the patient's perineum, the tip will be palpable during perineal exploration with the Haygrove sound. The use of the Haygrove staff is preferred at our institution, the staff merely being a circle-shaped sound. At other centers, other shapes of sound are preferred. If the tip of the scope is not felt, it may not be easily palpable during the dissection. In those cases, the authors create a temporary open vesicostomy to allow direct vision or palpation of the bladder neck, thus avoiding possible false passage or misanastomoses of the anterior urethra to sites other than the apical proximal urethra. Alternatively, the surgeon may use a flexible cystoscope and the Gelman-Haygrove staff later in the procedure. The Gelman staff is merely a circular-shaped, hollow sound, which allows for the flexible cystoscope to be placed through it. This then allows visual placement of the staff. The suprapubic catheter is then replaced and put to gravity drainage during the surgery.

The authors' technique is to place the patient in the exaggerated lithotomy position before surgery begins. The position is safe and provides excellent exposure to the membranous urethra and the prostatic apex (Fig. 6) [15,16]. Others employ the low lithotomy position with equal efficacy.

A custom table, modified to allow easy placement of the patient into the exaggerated lithotomy position, is helpful and shortens positioning time. The feet and legs are carefully positioned in the Guardian-style stirrups and protected with gel pads. The authors ensure proper positioning to avoid pressure on any part of the lower legs (Fig. 7). In addition, inward boot rotation is avoided. Such rotation can cause stretch injuries of the peroneal nerve (Fig. 8). The hips are elevated by raising the buttocks portion of the table. A solid gel roll is placed under the lumbar spine to support the forced kyphotic position. The lower extremities are suspended by the patient's feet within the boots of the stirrups.

Surgical technique aspects

The authors prefer an inverted lambda-shaped incision, which is outlined on the perineum (Fig. 6). Dissection is sharply carried through

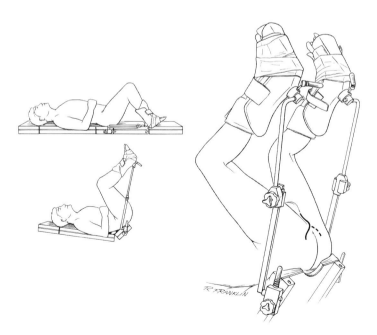

Fig. 6. Technique of placing a patient in the exaggerated lithotomy position. (*From* Angermeier KW, Jordan GH. Complications of exaggerated lithotomy position: a review of 177 cases. J Urol 1994:151:866–8.)

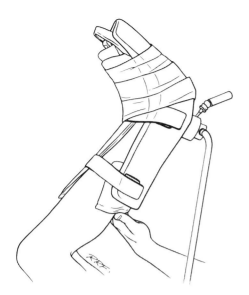

Fig. 7. Patient's legs in Guardian-style boots. No pressure should be placed on the calves or lower legs. (*From* Angermeier KW, Jordan GH. Complications of the exaggerated lithotomy position: a review of 177 cases. J Urol 1994;151:866–8.)

the subcutaneous tissue layers to the midline fusion of the ischiocavernosus muscles, remaining anterior to the transverse perineal musculature (ie, anterior perineal triangle) (Fig. 9). This approach is in contrast to that used for perineal prostatectomy, which is posterior to the transverse musculature (ie, posterior perineal triangle). Dissection continues distally along the ischiocavernosus muscle, revealing the uninvested portion of the corpus spongiosum. At this time, a self-retaining ring retractor is positioned. A number of table-fixed perineal retractors are available, and all are essential to facilitate surgical exposure.

The midline of the ischiocavernosus muscle is detached from the underlying corpus spongiosum (Fig. 9). The corpus spongiosum is then detached from the underlying corporal bodies and triangular ligament. The dissection is carried to the infrapubic space. Thus, the bulbospongiosus remains attached only by the fibrosis at the level of the distraction defect.

The arteries of the bulb and circumflex cavernosal arteries may be encountered lateral to the fibrotic zone. Often, the initial injury has obliterated these vessels. If found, the vessels are controlled with cautery. The authors avoid suture ligation in this region because of the potential proximity to the cavernous nerves. Dissection continues through the fibrotic band, dividing the

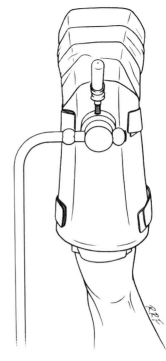

Fig. 8. Legs positioned in the Guardian-style stirrups. The boots must keep the lower legs in alignment to avoid stretch injury to the common peroneal nerve. (*From* Angermeier KW, Jordan GH. Complications of the exaggerated lithotomy position: a review of 177 cases. J Urol 1994;151:866–8.)

proximal point of the bulbous urethra (Fig. 9). At this point, the corpus spongiosum is mobilized distally somewhat.

Several steps can be followed to shorten the course of the anterior urethra. The first step is to divide the triangular ligament and develop the intracrural space (Fig. 10). The plane between the corporal bodies is often apparent. Occasionally, crossing vessels run transversally between the corpora and can be controlled with bipolar cautery and divided if necessary. Before dividing any vessel, determine that these are not the dorsal penile arteries, which may have been displaced medially at the time of the trauma. If in doubt, Doppler can be used. Dissection through the intracrural space reveals the undersurface of the deep dorsal vein of the penis. This vessel can be ligated and divided, usually revealing the tissues against the pubic bone. These maneuvers are usually adequate to produce sufficient shortening of the course of the anterior urethra for a tension-free anastomosis and for improving the exposure. If the course of the anterior urethra is not short enough, the

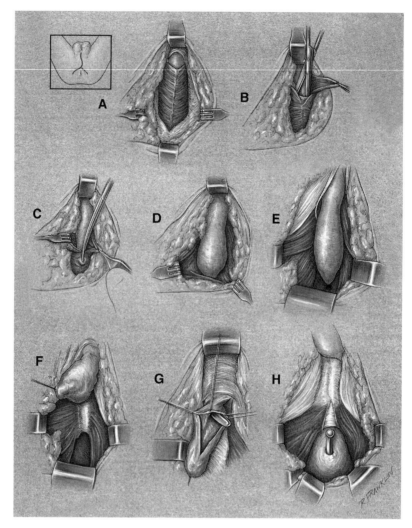

Fig. 9. Mobilizing the corpus spongium. (*A*) The midline fusion of the ischiocavernosus musculature is exposed. (*B,C,D*) The musculature is dissected from the bulbospongiosum. (*E*) The corpus spongiosum detached from the triangular ligament and the corpora cavernosa, remains attached proximally only by the fibrosis of the distraction defect. (*F*) The area of fibrosis is divided. (*G*) The anterior urethra is spatulated on its dorsal aspect. (*H*) The fibrosis is excised and the posterior urethrotomy spatulated. (*From* Walsh PC, Retik AB, Stamey TA, et al. Campbell's urology, 6th edition. Philadelphia: WB Saunders; 1992.)

corpus spongiosum is mobilized more vigorously out to, but not beyond, the plane of the penopubic attachments.

After the suprapubic tube has been removed, the Haygrove sound is passed through the suprapubic sinus tract or temporary vesicostomy and through the bladder neck to the point of obliteration. The impulse of the sound should be palpable within the fibrosis where the anterior urethra was detached. The fibrotic tissue overlying the sound is sequentially excised until the tip of the

instrument is concealed only by normal appearing urethral epithelium. The urethral epithelium is incised and controlled with temporary sutures. Endoscopy is performed through the urethrotomy to confirm that the sound has passed through the bladder neck and prostatic urethra and that the subsequent anastomosis will be at the most distal point of the healthy posterior urethra.

If the impulse of the sound is not palpable within the fibrotic tissue despite appropriate guidance of the sound down through the bladder

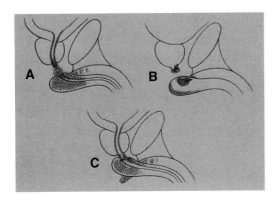

Fig. 10. (*A–C*) Posterior urethral anastomosis employing mobilization of the corpus spongiosum with development of the intracrural space.

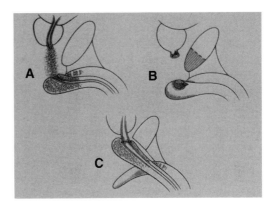

Fig. 12. Posterior urethral anatomosis. (*A*) Mobilization of the corpus spongiosum. (*B*) Extensive infrapubectomy. (*C*) Rerouting of the corpus spongiosum.

neck, then the posterior urethra and the sound are probably displaced behind the pubis. In this case, infrapubectomy is necessary to expose the distal posterior urethra (Fig. 11).

Rarely, the proximal urethra may be so rostrally distracted that infrapubectomy and corporal separation fails to adequately shorten the path of the anterior urethra. In such cases, the anterior urethra is rerouted around the corporal body to reduce the distance to the proximal stump (Fig. 12). A tunnel is created along the soft tissue surrounding the corporal body, with careful dissection avoiding the neurovascular bundle that is closely applied to its surface. Further osteotomy prevents urethral compression as the corpus spongiosum now courses between the corporal body and the pubis. Urethral reroute is seldom necessary in the authors' experience, but others frequently employ it [17].

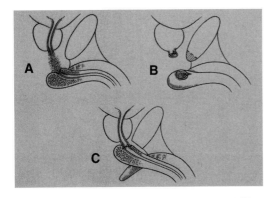

Fig. 11. Posterior urethral anastomosis. (*A*) Mobilization of the corpus spongiosum. (*B*) Development of the intracrural space. (*C*) Infrapubectomy.

After employing these maneuvers, a tension-free anastomosis should be guaranteed. The proximal urethrotomy is widely spatulated, with attention not to strip the fragile mucosa. Ten to 12 proximal anastomotic sutures are placed circumferentially, incorporating epithelium and surrounding connective tissue for support. The authors use alternating 3-0 or 4-0 polydioxanone and 3-0 or 4-0 Monocryl sutures.

The proximal bulbous urethra is spatulated to approximately 30 F on its dorsal surface and the anastomotic sutures are sequentially placed but not seated. The anterior urethra is delivered toward the posterior urethra, and slack is taken out of the anastomotic sutures. Before seating the anastomosis, the authors introduce a 14 F silicone (eg, Silastic) urethral stenting catheter through the anastomosis under direct vision. After the anastomosis is complete, the corpus spongiosum is reanchored to the corporal bodies. The bulbospongiosus musculature is approximated in the midline using interrupted sutures, with a suction drain placed deep to the muscle closure. The Colles' fascia is reapproximated and another suction drain is placed superficial to it. Both drains exit separately in the inguinoscrotal region. The skin is approximated using absorbable sutures. The authors use transparent adhesive dressing over the perineal closure. The urethral stent is plugged and the cystostomy tube is connected to gravity drainage.

Postoperative care

The patient is kept in bed for 24 to 48 hours and allowed to ambulate after that period. Erect sitting is not advisable. The neurovascular status in the lower limbs is carefully checked. Compartment syndrome or rhabdomyolysis are rarely seen in patients who have been in the exaggerated lithotomy position for less than 5 hours [18].

Self-limited neurapraxia of the dorsum feet is almost always resolved within 48 hours.

Pneumatic antiembolic stockings are used until the patient ambulates. Erections are suppressed with diazepam and amyl nitrite, and bladder spasms are controlled with an oral antimuscarinics. Intravenous antibiotics are employed the first 2 days postoperatively, and then switched to suppressive therapy if the urine culture demonstrates sterile urine. The patient is discharged on postoperative day 3. The authors usually perform the voiding trial with contrast on approximately the 21st postoperative day. The suprapubic catheter can be removed a few days after the voiding trial, after having been plugged at the time of the voiding trial.

Urethral straddle injuries

Physiopathology and location of traumatic injuries to the anterior urethra

Straddle trauma to the urethra occurs because of blunt force applied to the perineum acting as a hammer against the pubis, which acts as an anvil. The blunt crushing forces injure the urethra in a variety of fashions, ranging from what amounts to a contusion of the corpus spongiosum with minimal injury to the epithelium, to outright disruption of the urethra with total crushing of the corpus spongiosum. As already mentioned, the location of the injury depends on the angle at which the patient strikes the astride structure. These injuries usually affect only a short portion of the urethra.

Clinical presentation, diagnosis, and initial management of straddle trauma to the urethra

Patients with straddle trauma present with the history of straddle injury. Blood at the meatus may or may not be seen. Localized perineal hematomas confined to the boundaries of Buck's fascia or the tunica dartos are often seen. If Buck's fascia is ruptured, then the hematoma will be limited only by the overlying tunica dartos or Colles' fascia (Fig. 13). In most cases, the patient cannot void. In some cases, the patient can void but with considerable dysuria. The authors recommend that blind insertion of a urethral

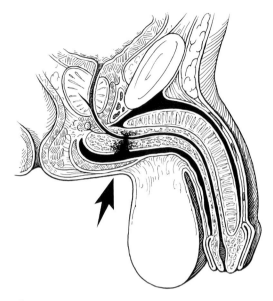

Fig. 13. Fall-astride injury to the perineum. In most cases, the Buck's fascia is disrupted. Often these patients present with the characteristic butterfly hematoma. Arrow shows point of insertion of the tunica dartos and Colles' fascia.

catheter be avoided. It is, however, safe to employ an endoscope with these patients, and in many cases a urethral catheter can be inserted. In these cases, the catheter can initially serve as the diversion. In the authors' opinion, the urethral catheter may serve as a drain, thus limiting the occurrence of infection of the perineal hematoma. Such infections can lead to periurethral abscess, which is frequently encountered with these injuries. It is the normal practice of the authors, in cases of complete disruption of the urethra, to also place a suprapubic catheter. In these cases, blunt suprapubic catheter placement can be accomplished. This approach differs from the preferred approach in the case of a pelvic fracture urethral distraction defect.

Diagnosis and initial management of the straddle injury

A retrograde urethrogram is the standard method for diagnosing these straddle injuries. If the watertight continuity of the urethra has been disturbed, the surgeon will see extravasation. In the cases of contusion of the corpus spongiosum with possible injury to the urethral epithelium, the surgeon can appreciate the mass effect of the intracorpus spongiosal hematoma. The authors

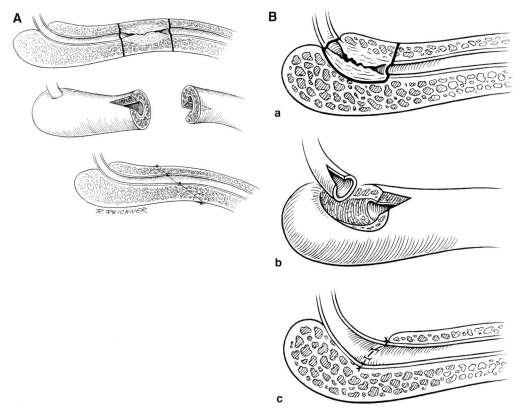

Fig. 14. (*A*) Technique for primary urethral anastomosis. In the midbulbous urethra, a two-layered spatulated anastomosis is preferred. (*From* Jordan GH. Principles of plastic surgery. In: Droller MJ, editor. Surgical management of urologic disease: an anatomic approach. Philadelphia: Mosby-Yearbook; 1992. p. 1218–37.) (*B*) Technique for primary urethral anastomosis. If the stricture is proximate to the departure of the bulbous urethra from the membranous urethra, then a single-layer spatulated anastomosis is performed. (*From* Jordan GH. Schlossberg SM. Chapter 110. Surgery of the penis and urethra. In: Campbell's urology, 8th edition. Walsh PC, Retik AB, Vaughan ED Jr, et al, editors. Philadelphia: WB Saunders; 2002, p. 3886–954.)

normally use an endoscope in these cases. If evidence suggests urethral epithelial injury, then diversion via a Foley catheter is accomplished. In these cases, the authors do not favor immediate repair because it is often difficult to determine the precise limits of the crush injury.

The repair is usually delayed for at least 3 months from the date of trauma. If the patient develops a perineal abscess, the repair may be further delayed.

Surgery for straddle injury urethral strictures

After resolution of the acute event, patients are carefully studied with a combination of retrograde and voiding urethrogram to determine the precise anatomy of the defect. In many cases where the urethra has been completely severed, the urethral lumen has been obliterated. Endoscopic procedures, such as dilation or internal urethrotomy, are seldom curative. Also, a urethral stent in cases of fall-astride perineal trauma is seldom useful. The resulting strictures are usually narrow caliber, short length, and can be repaired by a perineal approach. The gold standard treatment is excision with primary anastomosis. Several medical centers report success rates in excess of 95%. If the defect is somewhat longer, then an augmented anastomotic technique can be employed.

One-stage perineal anastomotic repair of the membranous urethra

For one-stage perineal anastomotic repairs of the membranous urethra, preoperative and early surgical steps are the same as those described for posterior urethral management. Complete exposure of the corpus spongiosum can be difficult in some cases of straddle trauma because the crush injury can obliterate the anatomy considerably. However the entire bulbous urethra must be dissected and exposed. In many cases, a significant length remains of proximal bulbous urethra, and in these cases the proximal blood supply must be protected from injury. However, if the anterior urethra is transected at its departure from the membranous urethra, the vessels can be divided.

After the stricture is localized and debridement is completed, both urethral ends are spatulated and an overlapped mucosa-to-mucosa anastomosis is performed over a 14 F catheter (Figs. 14A and 14B). The authors generally employ a suprapubic catheter. The anastomosis is a two-layer anastomosis if done in the more distal bulbous urethra or a single-layer anastomosis if done at the bulbo-membranous junction. As in the case of pelvic fracture urethral distraction defects, the development of the intracrural space can limit the need to mobilize the corpus spongiosum. However, infrapubectomy and rerouting are not a consideration as displacement rostrally of the proximal urethra is not present in these injuries. The wound is drained and closed as already mentioned.

Drains are placed under the muscle plane and superficial to the perineum. They are usually removed on postoperative day 2 or 3.

Postoperative care

The patient is admitted typically for 2 to 3 days, and kept on bed rest for 24 to 36 hours. Upright sitting is restricted to limit pressure on the mobilized corpus spongiosum.

Prophylactic broad-spectrum antibiotics are discontinued 24 to 48 hours after surgery and the patient is switched to suppressive antibiotics until the suprapubic tube is removed. The patient is discharged with a suprapubic tube connected to continuous drainage and a urethral catheter plugged. The last is removed in the office after 2 to 3 weeks and a voiding cystourethrogram is done. The suprapubic catheter is removed 3 to 4 days later if the patient voids without difficulty.

Summary

While traumatic injuries to the urethra can have devastating consequences, successful reconstruction is possible in most cases. The issues of erectile dysfunction often plague the patient long term. However, these patients are rarely limited by the urethral stricture process per se. Endoscopic procedures seldom cure these lesions. Also, indwelling stents are seldom useful in these cases. In cases where stents have been inserted, a process that normally could be readily repaired with a primary anastomotic technique often becomes a more involved process that requires tubed reconstruction of the urethra. Primary anastomotic techniques are associated with success rates in the high 90% range and are felt to be durable for most cases. In contrast, tubed reconstruction of the urethra is inevitably associated with diminished success rates and with problems of durability.

References

 [1] Aboseif SR, Breza J, Lue TF, et al. Penile venous drainage in erectile dysfunction: anatomical, radiological and functional considerations. Br J Urol 1989;64:183–90.
 [2] Pokorny M, Pontes E, Pierce JM Jr. Urological injuries associated with pelvic trauma. J Urol 1979;121: 455.
 [3] Colapinto V, McCallum RM. Injury to the male posterior urethra in fractured pelvis: a new classification. J Urol 1977;118:575–80.
 [4] Goldman SM, Sandler CM, Corriere JM, et al. Blunt urethra trauma: a unified, anatomical mechanical classification. J Urol 1997;157(1):85–9.
 [5] Chapple C, Barbagli G, Jordan GH, et al. Consensus statement on urethral trauma. Br J Urol 2004;93: 1195–202.
 [6] Mouraviev VB, Santucci RA. Cadaveric anatomy of pelvic fracture urethral distraction injury: most injuries are distal to the external urinary sphincter. J Urol 2005;173:869–72.
 [7] Andrich DE, Mundy AR. The nature of urethral injury in cases of pelvic fracture urethral trauma. J Urol 2001;165(5):1492–5.
 [8] Andrich DE, O'Malley KJ, Summerton DJ, et al. The type of urethroplasty for a pelvic fracture urethral distraction defect cannot be predicted preoperatively. J Urol 2003;170(2 Pt1):464–7.
 [9] Ziran BH, Chamberlin E, Shuler FD, et al. Delays and difficulties in the diagnosis of lower urologic injuries in the context of pelvic fractures. J Trauma 2005;58:533–7.
[10] McCoy GB, Barry JM, Lieberman SF, et al. Treatment of obliterated membraneous and bulbous urethras by direct vision internal urethrotomy. J Trauma 1987;27(8):883–6.
[11] Young HH. Treatment of complete rupture of the posterior urethra, recent or ancient, by anastomosis. J Urol 1929;21:417.

[12] Badenoch AWA. Pull-through operation for impassable traumatic stricture of the urethra. Br J Urol 1950;22(4):404–9.

[13] Iselin CE, Webster GD. The significance of the open bladder neck associated with pelvic fracture urethral distraction defects. J Urol 1999;162:34–51.

[14] Waterhouse K, Abrahams JI, Gruber H, et al. The transpubic approach to the lower urinary tract. J Urol 1973;109:486–90.

[15] Angermeier KW, Jordan GH. Complications of the exaggerated lithotomy position: A review of 177 cases. J Urol 1994;151 966–868.

[16] Miller KS, Lee-Quen P, Pranikoff K, et al. Neurologic complications of the exaggerated lithotomy position during urethral reconstructive surgery: a prospective study. J Urol, submitted for publication.

[17] Webster GD, Mathes GL, Selli C. Prostatomembranous urethral injuries: a review of the literature and a rational approach to their management. J Urol 1983;130:898–902.

[18] Anema JG, Morey AF, McAninch JW, et al. Complications related to the high lithotomy position during urethral reconstruction. J Urol 2000;164: 360–3.

ELSEVIER
SAUNDERS

Urol Clin N Am 33 (2006) 111–116

UROLOGIC
CLINICS
of North America

Diagnosis and Management of Testicular Ruptures

Jill C. Buckley, MD[a,b], Jack W. McAninch, MD[a,b,*]

[a]Department of Urology, University of California School of Medicine, San Francisco, CA, USA
[b]Urology Service, 3A20, San Francisco General Hospital, 1001 Potrero Avenue, San Francisco, CA 94110, USA

Testicular trauma most commonly occurs in young men between the ages of 15 and 40 years. There are serious repercussions if a testicular rupture is missed. Although not life threatening, loss of a testicle could impair future fertility, contribute to a hypogonal state, and affect social confidence. These patients present with scrotal trauma often accompanied by a difficult clinical examination because of a swollen, tender, ecchymotic scrotum. With the high incidence of testicular ruptures associated with scrotal trauma, early diagnosis and operative intervention are critical to achieve high salvage rates.

Ultrasonography has become an extension of the clinical examination in assessing the integrity of the testicle in scrotal trauma. Focusing on the single radiographic finding of a heterogeneous echopattern of the testicular parenchyma with a loss of contour definition, ultrasonography has demonstrated a sensitivity and specificity of ≥95% in diagnosing testicular ruptures [1].

The goal in evaluating scrotal trauma is prompt diagnosis of a testicular rupture to allow timely operative exploration and reconstruction. Early diagnosis and intervention lead to high testicular salvage rates [1,2]. Both penetrating and blunt scrotal trauma can lead to a testicular rupture. With rare exception, penetrating trauma to the scrotum is explored, yielding few missed injuries and allowing immediate repair. Blunt trauma presents more of a diagnostic dilemma because immediate operative exploration is

not necessarily indicated. A difficult scrotal examination can prevent detection of a testicular rupture, an oversight that can have severe repercussions.

In the early 1980s, Cass and coworkers [3,4] reported a high incidence of testicular rupture (45%) in blunt scrotal trauma and championed early operative exploration for all scrotal trauma to decrease the incidence of delayed orchiectomy. With early exploration now the standard of care, the challenge lies in prompt diagnosis and successful reconstruction. Many centers, including San Francisco General Hospital (SFGH), rely on ultrasonography to determine management when the clinical examination is nondiagnostic. Based on a 25-year experience with blunt scrotal trauma (the largest series to date), the authors reported the incidence, diagnosis, and management of testicular injuries and demonstrated the use of scrotal ultrasonography. With a prompt diagnosis based on a reliable clinical examination, or scrotal ultrasonography after inconclusive examination, they achieved a testicular rupture salvage rate of 83% [1].

Initial presentation

Most testicular ruptures are a result of blunt trauma and are initially seen by an urgent care or emergency department physician. Immediately, the mechanism of injury can be determined as either blunt or penetrating to direct the initial management. With rare exception, penetrating trauma to the scrotum needs to be operatively explored [5]. Under anesthesia a thorough testicular examination can be performed, followed by operative exploration of the testis if the integrity of the tunica albuginea is in question or a large expanding hematoma is encountered.

* Corresponding author. Urology Service, 3A20, San Francisco General Hospital, 1001 Potrero Avenue, San Francisco, CA 94110.
E-mail address: jmcaninch@urol.ucsf.edu (J.W. McAninch).

Unlike penetrating trauma to the scrotum, not all blunt scrotal trauma requires an operation. In the series at SFGH, 44 (68%) of the 65 patients underwent operative exploration. Thirty (68%) of the 44 patients were explored for testicular rupture, consistent with the other large series in the literature [2]. Common etiologies, such as motor vehicles accident, falls, and sport-related injuries (Table 1), create a difficult clinical examination that cannot adequately assess the integrity of the testicle. Because the scrotum is an elastic and distensible space, significant swelling or bleeding can occur, dramatically distorting the normal anatomy. To avoid operative exploration in every patient presenting with scrotal trauma and a nondiagnostic clinical examination, scrotal ultrasonography has emerged as the study of choice for testicular evaluation with excellent sensitivity and specificity. In the SFGH experience of 65 patients presenting with blunt scrotal trauma, 53 (82%) had associated testicular or peritesticular injuries consisting of contusions, hematoceles, testicular dislocations, intratesticular hematomas, and testicular ruptures. Tunica albuginea rupture was present in 30 (46%); all were unilateral. With testicular rupture present in >40% of all blunt scrotal trauma, it must be actively screened for with a diagnostic physical examination or scrotal ultrasonography [1,6].

Diagnosis

A testicular rupture is defined as a rupture of the tunica albuginea with protrusion of the seminiferous tubules. Penetrating scrotal trauma is immediately explored. A thorough examination under anesthesia is accompanied by direct inspection of the tunica albuginea if the integrity of the testicle is in question.

Most scrotal trauma is the result of blunt injury. In some of these patients, the clinical examination alone is definitive enough to determine

Table 1
Mechanism of blunt scrotal injuries (65 patients)

Assault	33%
Motor vehicle accident	22%
Athletic injuries	8.5%
Falls	8.5%
Other	22%

Data from Buckley JC, McAninch JW. Use of ultrasonography for the diagnosis of testicular injuries in blunt scrotal trauma. J Urol 2006;175:175–8; with permission.

management. For the remaining cases, scrotal ultrasonography has emerged as the imaging modality of choice to assess the state of the testis and the surrounding tissue. The major physical finding suggesting testicular rupture is extreme testicular tenderness and pain during palpation. In the SFGH blunt scrotal trauma series, preoperative scrotal ultrasonography was performed in 47 of 65 patients in whom the integrity of the testicle could not be accurately assessed by clinical examination alone. Operative exploration was undertaken in 32 patients with radiographic findings positive for testicular rupture: heterogeneous echo pattern of the testicular parenchyma with loss of contour definition. With improved technology, real-time high-resolution ultrasound has provided an accurate window into the viability of the internal scrotal structures despite external swelling and ecchymosis. Using the 7.5-MHz transverse probe, contusions, hematoceles, testicular dislocations, intratesticular hematomas, and testicular ruptures can be visualized. The size, consistency of the parenchyma, relation to surrounding structures, and comparison with the contralateral side can greatly assist in the initial evaluation, diagnosis, and management of a testicular rupture [7–10].

Ultrasonographic diagnosis of testicular rupture

The diagnosis of testicular rupture is based on the single radiographic finding of a heterogeneous echo pattern of the testicular parenchyma with a loss of contour definition (Fig. 1A). Historically, fracture of tunica albuginea was the criteria used to diagnose a testicular rupture using ultrasonography; however, this has since been shown to have poor sensitivity and specificity and no longer guides management [11,12]. In the authors' series, 32 patients were explored for sonographic findings consistent with a testicular rupture. Thirty were confirmed intraoperatively, for a specificity of 93.5%. The two false-positives (a true-positive was defined as a rupture of the tunica albuginea), were an intratesticular hematoma and a testicular contusion, both demonstrated an intact tunica albuginea. Scrotal ultrasonography proved to be 100% sensitive, as no delayed orchiectomy was required for an undetected testicular rupture in those patients with normal radiographic results. In patients who have a radiographically normal, homogeneous-appearing testicle, no exploration is necessary. Doppler imaging of the testicle is not routinely performed.

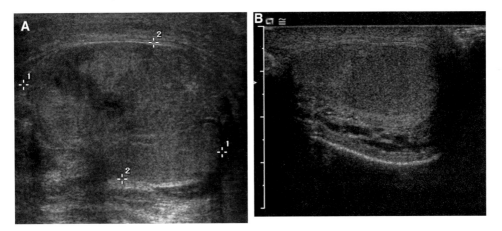

Fig. 1. Scrotal ultrasonography of a blunt testicular rupture. (*A*) Preoperatively. Note the very heterogeneous echo pattern of the testicular parenchyma. (*B*) Postoperatively. Excellent preservation of parenchyma with a homogeneous appearance.

Operative management

Most testicular ruptures can be reconstructed primarily. In the authors' experience at SFGH, 24 of 25 cases occurring from blunt trauma were primarily repaired, with the remaining patient requiring a free graft of the tunica vaginalis for coverage of the exposed testicular parenchyma. After the patient has been appropriately evaluated for other nonurologic injuries and stabilized, operative exploration of the scrotum can be performed. General anesthesia and gram-positive intravenous antibiotic coverage are given and a transverse incision is made in the lower third of scrotum over the injured testis. After opening the tunica vaginalis the testis is delivered to allow complete inspection of the tunica albuginea. The rupture site is easily identified with extruded seminiferous tubules (Fig. 2A). Sharp debridement of the necrotic, nonviable tissue is performed until healthy bleeding edges are encountered (Fig. 2B). The remaining tunica albuginea is closed with a small absorbable suture in a continuous fashion (Fig. 2C). The testis is placed back into the scrotum in its natural lie and a two-layer closure of the scrotum is performed with absorbable suture [5]. A penrose drain is placed through a separate incision to minimize swelling and typically is removed on postoperative day 2. Icing, elevation, and anti-inflammatory medication are immediately used. The patient is seen 2 weeks after discharge for a postoperative wound examination followed by a scrotal ultrasound at 3 months to evaluate healing.

Orchiectomy is reserved for critically ill patients with complex traumatic injuries where testicular reconstruction is not a life-saving priority.

Delayed operative exploration

Unlike a testicular torsion where the arterial blood supply is completely compromised requiring immediate exploration, a testicular rupture is a relative ischemic state. In the SFGH series, 5 of 30 blunt trauma testicular ruptures presented >3 days after the initial insult, the authors' definition of a delayed presentation. Although only one out of five underwent testicular reconstruction, the authors believe every testicular rupture should be approached with the intent to salvage the testicle. After thorough operative exploration, if the testicle is clearly unsalvageable an orchiectomy should be performed.

Nonoperative management

It is the authors' opinion that there is no role for nonoperative management of testicular ruptures. Operative exploration and reconstruction should be performed to preserve hormonal function and maintain parenchymal volume, and to prevent abscess formation and chronic pain which often results in orchiectomy.

Discussion

Penetrating scrotal trauma is explored expediting the diagnosis and reconstruction of testicular

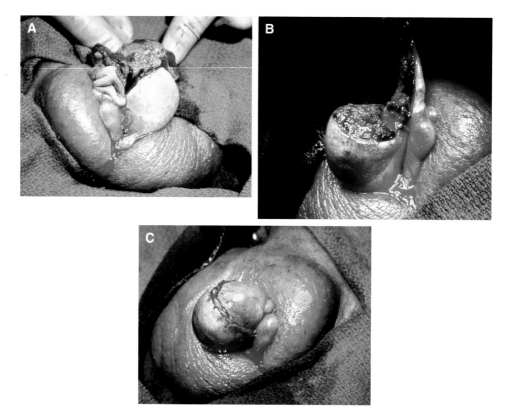

Fig. 2. (*A*) Intraoperative view of testicular rupture with extruded seminiferous tubule. (*B, C*) Testicular repair consisting of debridement and primary tunical closure.

ruptures. Before 1968, blunt scrotal trauma was managed conservatively, often without hospitalization; thus, the incidence of testicular rupture was unknown. A dramatic shift in patient care occurred in the 1970s from a watch-and-wait approach to today's standard of early operative exploration and reconstruction (Cass [3] and Gross' [13] 20-year experiences). They compared primary conservative management (testicular ruptures before 1971) with early operative exploration and repair [3]. They found a 45% orchiectomy rate in the delayed surgical intervention group (primary conservative management) versus a 9% orchiectomy rate in the early surgical exploration group (defined as within 3 days of the injury). This is the basis for management of testicular ruptures today.

In the series from SFGH focusing on blunt scrotal trauma, the overall operative scrotal exploration rate was 68%. Of these explorations, ≥65% were for testicular ruptures, with the remaining third performed for primary debridement,

drainage of hematoma, and scrotal skin closure or active bleeding. Clearly, a large number of blunt scrotal traumas require early operative intervention, specifically those that involve a ruptured testicle, to achieve a high salvage rate. Determining which case needs immediate exploration remains the challenge. In the setting of a tender or severely distorted scrotum, palpation of the testicles is virtually impossible; thus, one is left to look for other, more sensitive, diagnostic modalities [14]. At many institutions, including SFGH, scrotal ultrasonography has been found to be a highly sensitive and specific diagnostic tool to help guide management of blunt scrotal trauma. In the past, ultrasonography was far less sensitive, with a high false-negative rate [11,12], the direct result of its inability to document clearly the integrity of the tunica albuginea. At SFGH, the authors rely on the single radiographic finding of a heterogeneous echo pattern of the testicular parenchyma with a loss of contour definition (see Fig. 1A), and they do not attempt to identify a fracture of the tunica albuginea.

This avoids false-negative findings, dramatically improving the sensitivity of ultrasonography while maintaining specificity [1,10,15].

The scrotal ultrasound can be performed by the "on-call" radiologist and interpreted concurrently with the urologist. At SFGH, it was found to be a reliable and reproducible examination. The authors believe that by focusing on this single criterion, urologists can accurately diagnose a testicular rupture.

Immediate operative exploration and repair are imperative for testicular salvage. A delay in diagnosis leads to an unacceptably high orchiectomy rate [3]. Once exploration is undertaken, very attempt should be made to salvage the remaining viable testicular tissue with debridement and primary reconstruction [5]. A small study compared semen analysis parameters between men who underwent primary testicular reconstruction and orchiectomy for testicular ruptures. They concluded the testicular salvage group had no significant seminal or endocrine abnormalities, whereas the orchiectomy group demonstrated a significant decrease in sperm density and elevation of baseline follicle-stimulating hormone and luteinizing hormone. This supports an aggressive attempt at testicular reconstruction over orchiectomy even in the setting of a severe testicular rupture with a normal contralateral testis [16]. This may seem unlikely (see Fig. 2A), but with complete exposure of the tunica albuginea and debridement of the extruded seminiferous tubules a surprising amount of the testicle can be salvaged (see Fig. 2B). Other benefits of early operative exploration and repair are a quicker resolution of pain, control of bleeding, a theoretical prevention of antisperm antibodies, and preservation of spermatogenesis. Patients require shorter hospital stays and return sooner to daily activities [2,17].

The authors' experience included one patient with a solitary testicle who suffered a testicular rupture requiring exploration and repair. Both testicular volume and hormonal function were maintained at the 12-week follow-up visit. Albeit an isolated event, this suggests that immediate exploration and repair can preserve testicular parenchyma and its function because of the testicle's remarkable ability to heal. Fig. 1 shows the preoperative and postoperative scrotal ultrasound after primary repair of a testicular rupture with excellent preservation of the testicular parenchyma and a normal homogeneous appearance. This experience is consistent with reports of patients who undergo testicular sperm harvesting with excellent postoperative testicular parenchymal and hormonal preservation [18].

Equally important, but more difficult to quantify, is the psychologic benefit of testicular preservation for cosmesis. The reconstructed testicle maintains adequate testicular volume preventing a grossly abnormal physical appearance and the transverse scrotal incision is virtually undetectable after complete healing.

Without question, testicular ruptures need to be explored, debrided, and reconstructed, but that does not hold true for peritesticular injuries not directly involving a rupture. This gray area is controversial and often surgeon-dependent. Some argue that all testicular contusions resulting in a hematocele should be explored for earlier resolution of pain, shorter hospital stays, and an earlier return to daily activity [14,17]. At SFGH, because of the risks associated with anesthesia, surgery, and infection, every hematocele is not routinely explored, but rather its initial size and dynamics are determined. A large (>5 cm) or expanding scrotal hematoma is explored. If it is ≤ 5 cm and not actively enlarging, the authors often opt for conservative management consisting of elevation, scrotal support, nonsteroidal anti-inflammatory medication, icing, and pain control. When the hematoma is small and not expanding, the authors believe the integrity of the natural skin barrier is important in preventing infection, especially when access to proper hygiene may be unavailable. No patient required delayed drainage for a nonresolving hematoma. Additionally, no delayed orchiectomies were performed in this series (chronic pain from missed testicular rupture was the primary reason for delayed orchiectomy in Cass's [3] original work), supporting the belief that ultrasonography based on the authors' single radiographic criterion is extremely sensitive and prevents missing testicular ruptures. This results in a higher testicular salvage rate while minimizing unnecessary scrotal exploration.

Summary

Early diagnosis and operative reconstruction of a testicular rupture from either penetrating or blunt trauma can achieve high testicular salvage rates. Aggressive testicular preservation and reconstruction has hormonal, reproductive, and cosmetic benefits for the patient. A delay in diagnosis should not occur as penetrating injuries are explored and difficult blunt trauma scrotal examinations are supplemented with a sensitive and specific scrotal sonogram. In scrotal trauma, it is the responsibility of the physician to actively screen for testicular ruptures. With prompt diagnosis, debridement, and reconstruction high testicular salvage rates can be achieved avoiding the delayed complications of chronic pain, atrophy, and orchiectomy associated with missed testicular rupture.

References

[1] Buckley JC, McAninch JW. Use of ultrasonography for the diagnosis of testicular injuries in blunt scrotal trauma. J Urol 2006;175:175–8.

[2] Altarac S. Management of 53 cases of testicular trauma. Eur Urol 1994;25:119.

[3] Cass AS. Testicular trauma. J Urol 1983;129:299.

[4] Cass AS, Ferrara L, Wolpert J, et al. Bilateral testicular injury from external trauma. J Urol 1988;140: 1435.

[5] McAninch JW. Reconstruction of testicular rupture. In: Traumatic and reconstructive urology. Philadelphia: WB Saunders; 1996. p. 733–6.

[6] Barthelemy Y, Delmas V, Villers A, et al. Scrotal trauma: report of 33 cases. Prog Urol 1992;2:628.

[7] McAninch JW. Sonography in the staging of testicular trauma. In: Traumatic and reconstructive urology. Philadelphia: WB Saunders; 1996. p. 727–32.

[8] Pace A, Powell C. Testicular infarction and rupture after blunt trauma: use of diagnostic ultrasound. ScientificWorldJournal 2004;4:437.

[9] Patil MG, Onuora VC. The value of ultrasound in the evaluation of patients with blunt scrotal trauma. Injury 1994;25:177.

[10] Anderson KA, McAninch JW, Jeffrey RB, et al. Ultrasonography for the diagnosis and staging of blunt scrotal trauma. J Urol 1983;130:933.

[11] Corrales JG, Corbel L, Cipolla B, et al. Accuracy of ultrasound diagnosis after blunt testicular trauma. J Urol 1993;150:1834.

[12] Ugarte R, Spaedy M, Cass AS. Accuracy of ultrasound in diagnosis of rupture after blunt testicular trauma. Urology 1990;36:253.

[13] Gross M. Rupture of the testicle: the importance of early surgical treatment. J Urol 1969;101:196.

[14] Kratzik C, Hainz A, Kuber W, et al. Has ultrasound influenced the therapy concept of blunt scrotal trauma? J Urol 1989;142:1243.

[15] Jeffrey RB, Laing FC, Hricak H, et al. Sonography of testicular trauma. AJR Am J Roentgenol 1983; 141:993.

[16] Lin WW, Kim ED, Quesada ET, et al. Unilateral testicular injury from external trauma: evaluation of semen quality and endocrine parameters. J Urol 1998;159:841.

[17] Cass AS, Luxenberg M. Value of early operation in blunt testicular contusion with hematocele. J Urol 1988;139:746.

[18] Schill T, Bals-Pratsch M, Kupker W, et al. Clinical and endocrine follow-up of patients after testicular sperm extraction. Fertil Steril 2003;79:281.

ELSEVIER
SAUNDERS

Urol Clin N Am 33 (2006) 117–126

UROLOGIC
CLINICS
of North America

Penile and Genital Injuries

Hunter Wessells, MD, FACS*, Layron Long, MD

*Department of Urology, University of Washington School of Medicine and Harborview Medical Center,
325 Ninth Avenue, Seattle, WA 98104, USA*

Genital injuries are significant because of their association with injuries to major pelvic and vascular organs that result from both blunt and penetrating mechanisms, and the chronic disability resulting from penile, scrotal, and vaginal trauma. Because trauma is predominantly a disease of young persons, genital injuries may profoundly affect health-related quality of life and contribute to the burden of disease related to trauma. Injuries to the female genitalia have additional consequences because of the association with sexual assault and interpersonal violence [1]. Although the existing literature has many gaps, a recent Consensus Group on Genitourinary Trauma provided an overview and reference point on the subject [2]. This article reviews the mechanism, initial evaluation, and operative management of injuries to the male and female external genitalia including the penis, scrotal skin, and vaginal structures.

Prevalence

The incidence of genital injuries has not been determined, but in civilian centers is likely to be low, given that most case series span many years and include relatively small numbers of patients [3]. In the battlefield, the massive destruction caused by fragmentation devices, combined with the use of protective torso armor, has led to survival of soldiers with increasingly severe pelvic and genital organ injury [4]. Penile fracture is the most commonly described blunt injury to the penis, and over 1300 cases have been reported in the literature [5].

---

* Corresponding author.
E-mail address: wessells@u.washington.edu
(H. Wessells).

Mechanisms

The male genitalia have a tremendous capacity to resist injury. The flaccidity of the pendulous portion of the penis limits the transfer of kinetic energy during trauma. In contrast, the fixed portion of the genitalia (eg, the crura of the penis in relation to the pubic rami, and the female external genitalia in their similar relationships with these bony structures) are prone to blunt trauma from pelvic fracture or straddle injury. Similarly, the erect penis becomes more prone to injury because increases in pressure within the penis during bending rise exponentially when the penis is rigid (up to 1500 mm Hg) as opposed to flaccid [6]. Injury caused by missed intromission or manual attempts at detumescence can cause penile fracture [7]. Less severe bending injuries may still lead to long-term disability related to tunica albuginea disruption (Peyronie's disease) or arterial insufficiency. Firearms and missiles have an excess of kinetic energy, which overcomes the protective mechanisms of flaccidity.

Another characteristic of the male genitalia particularly pertinent to injury mechanisms is the looseness and laxity of genital skin. Although this generally has a protective role, allowing the skin to deform and slide away from a potential point of contact, in the case of machinery injury, rotating or suction devices can grab hold of a portion of the genital skin [8]. Laxity of skin becomes a liability because the entire penile and scrotal skin can be trapped and avulsed.

The vascular supply of the genitalia also predicts outcomes of other forms of injury, such as chemical, radiant, and infectious injury. Deep structures have multiple sources of arterial inflow. The penis derives a triple blood flow from the dorsal, cavernosal, and bulbourethral arteries. Ischemic loss of this organ because of injury is only seen with complete amputation or prolonged constriction injury. Likewise, the testis derives blood supply from the cremasteric, testicular, and vasal arteries. In cases of Fournier's gangrene neither of these organs is lost. Conversely the skin, although richly vascularized through multiple sources, receives its arterial perfusion from deeper fascial layers, and when these are affected by synergistic bacterial infection during Fournier's gangrene, total skin loss is inevitable. Because burns start superficially and progressively spread their damage down into deeper tissues in the opposite fashion from Fournier's gangrene, preservation of some portion of the vascular integrity of the skin is likely in most chemical and thermal burns.

A particularly unusual cause of penile injury is amputation, which is discussed separately because of its unique considerations [9,10]. When assault is the cause, appropriate police reporting is required. Other cases require special input from psychiatric and psychologic experts. Penile amputation may be a manifestation of depressive and psychotic behavior, either caused by schizophrenia or illicit drug abuse. Others amputate the penis to initiate the process of gender conversion. Finally, constriction rings can cause loss of superficial skin, deep urethral necrosis, or complete penile loss.

Blunt injuries cause much less damage to the phallus than firearm and stab injuries. The laxity of the genital skin usually protects the deep penile structures from avulsion, so that after car crashes superficial lacerations of the skin are more common. Pelvic fractures with symphyseal or pubic ramus displacement can cause severe injury to the deep structures of the penis, including avulsion of the crus of the corpus cavernosum from its vascular and neural supply [11]. Less severe crush injuries may also occur. The long-term consequences of these injuries are more significant than their initial presentation suggests. Although extensive bleeding may occur, angioembolization of the internal pudendal arterial tree can control such hemorrhage. More importantly, the delayed consequences of arterial injury are erectile dysfunction or penile ischemia. Tables 1 and 2 show the characteristics of injuries to the penis and scrotum, and corresponding AIS scores.

Presentation

Penetrating injuries to the external genitalia require special consideration because of the high

Table 1
Organ injury scale for penile injury

AAST grade	Penile injury	AIS-90 score
I	Cutaneous laceration or contusion	1
II	Laceration of Buck's fascia (cavernosum) without tissue loss	1
III	Cutaneous avulsion, laceration through glans or meatus, or cavernosal or urethral defect <2 cm	3
IV	Partial penectomy or cavernosal or urethral defect = 2 cm	3
V	Total penectomy	3

Abbreviations: AAST, American Association for the Surgery of Trauma; AIS, Abbreviated Injury Scale.

From Moore EE, Malangoni MA, Cogbill TH, et al. Organ injury scaling VII: cervical vascular, peripheral vascular, adrenal, penis, testis, and scrotum. J Trauma 1996;41:523; with permission.

likelihood of associated injuries to the spermatic cord and testis, urinary bladder and urethra, rectum, and vascular structures of the iliac and femoral region. Blood at the urethral meatus implies injury, whereas its absence can be misleading. Urethral injury occurs in 10% to 38% of penile fractures and up to 22% of penile gunshot wounds [12,13].

A delayed presentation is not uncommon after penile fracture and constriction ring use, usually caused by patient embarrassment. The constellation of missed intromission, acute bending, and

Table 2
AAST organ injury scale for scrotal injury

AAST grade	Scrotal injury	AIS-90 score
I	Contusion	1
II	Laceration <25% of scrotal diameter	1
III	Laceration = 25% of scrotal diameter	2
IV	Avulsion <50%	2
V	Avulsion = 50%	2

Abbreviations: AAST, American Association for the Surgery of Trauma; AIS, Abbreviated Injury Scale.

From Moore EE, Malangoni MA, Cogbill TH, et al. Organ injury scaling VII: cervical vascular, peripheral vascular, adrenal, penis, testis, and scrotum. J Trauma 1996;41:523; with permission.

a popping sound followed by immediate detumescence of the penis and acute pain are characteristic of this entity. In the Middle East and other regions, penile fracture may occur as a result of excessive bending of the shaft in an attempt to achieve rapid detumescence of an embarrassing penile erection [7]. Penile swelling is usually limited to the attachments of Buck's fascia and only the shaft of the penis is ecchymotic; a localized hematoma is evident in such cases and has been termed an "eggplant deformity" [2]. When the deep investing fascia of the penis has been ruptured by penetrating or blunt trauma, a perineal butterfly hematoma or scrotal bleeding can occur. Entrapment of the genitalia by industrial machinery including augers, power takeoff from farm tractors, and suction devices can lead to avulsion of the penile and scrotal skin (Fig. 1).

Genital and perineal burns are present in less than 5% of burn victims, and patients hospitalized for burns involve the genitalia and perineum [14].

Initial evaluation

The evaluation and initial management of genital injuries involves recognition of associated injuries, control of hemorrhage, and certain mechanism-specific interventions. Penetrating injuries to the penis have associated injuries in up to 83% of patients. Those with associated urethral injury usually present with blood at the urethral meatus and inability to void; the absence of these signs does not exclude urethral injury [2]. Retrograde urethrogram is the appropriate test for suspected urethral injuries caused by either penetrating or blunt injuries, in particular penile fracture. In the absence of obvious signs of urethral injury, urethral catheterization should be attempted before exploration and can help maintain

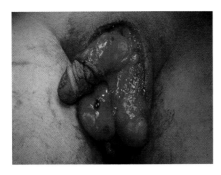

Fig. 1. Patient with scrotal and penile skin avulsion after pants were caught in posthole digger.

orientation when structures are distorted by hematoma. The presence of hematuria should alert the trauma team to the possibility of a bladder or upper urinary tract injury in cases of penetrating firearm injuries. Finally, rectal injuries must be sought out if complications, such as fistulae and Fournier's gangrene, are to be avoided.

Bleeding from the penis can usually be controlled in the emergency department with gauze wraps to tamponade any bleeding. Excessively tight compressive dressings that compromise blood supply to the distal penis must be avoided.

The mechanism of injury is important. Burns should be covered with appropriate dressings depending on the mechanism. For thermal injury, 1% silver sulfadiazine cream is appropriate. Chemical burns can be irrigated with saline; lye burns should not be irrigated with water, which can cause further caustic damage. For alkaline burns, dilute acetic acid should be used. For acid burns, sodium bicarbonate is recommended [15].

Bite injuries by animals or humans require appropriate antibiotic coverage for the species and tetanus toxoid administration [15]. Empirical broad-spectrum antibiotics, such as amoxicillin–clavulinic acid are appropriate for dog, rat, cat, bat, skunk, and raccoon bites and human bites. In cases of animal bites, the possibility of rabies transmission must be considered. Dog and cat bites most commonly lead to pathogenic infection with *Pasteurella* organisms; anaerobic organisms may also be present [16]. Many rare pathogens can be transmitted from dogs. Human bites are morel likely to cause complications than dog bite wounds. The predominant human oral bacterial organism is *Eikenella corrodens*; however, transmission of viral infection including hepatitis and HIV is possible [17].

After penile amputation or self-mutilation, appropriate experts must be involved to ascertain the competence of the patient and allow appropriate decision making when considering replantation of the penis. Urinary diversion should be established with a suprapubic cystostomy. The stump should be covered with compressive sterile saline-soaked gauze dressings. Bleeding can be extensive and transfusion may be required [2]. Once the patient has been resuscitated, surgical planning for replantation can continue. The amputated phallus is treated with a two-bag system [9]. In the inner bag, the amputated organ is wrapped in sterile saline gauze, and then the entire first bag is placed into a second bag containing ice. With this approach, appropriate transfer to tertiary centers can be accomplished with successful reimplantation over 24 hours after injury.

Cavernosography has been proposed as an adjunct to the diagnosis of penile fracture and may also have specific applications to cases of penetrating trauma [18]. Most cases require operative repair, however, and such ancillary tests, with limited sensitivity and specificity, are not clinically useful. If one repairs all penetrating and blunt ruptures of the tunica albuginea and superficial penile structures, radiographic studies of the corpora cavernosa are not necessary. Cavernosography, ultrasound, and MRI may be useful in selected cases to confirm that a penile fracture is absent and that a nonoperative approach is appropriate [2]. Once associated urethral, scrotal, bladder, and rectal injuries have been excluded or identified, then appropriate management of penile injuries can occur.

Operative management

The goal of surgery is to restore penile function and appearance. The operative repair of genital injuries involves appropriate irrigation, debridement, and closure of all wound layers, taking into account associated injuries that may influence treatment, the degree of contamination and tissue damage, and the time from injury to repair. For example, in the absence of gross contamination or delayed presentation, the presence of a rectal injury or even a human bite injury may not preclude an excellent functional and cosmetic outcome. Conversely, prioritization must take place in the face of multiple vascular or other organ injuries.

Exposure of the deep cavernosum and tunica albuginea can be achieved through either a circumferential subcoronal incision by degloving, or for deeper wounds a penoscrotal, infrapubic, or even perineal incision. For penile fracture, the injury occurs almost exclusively distal to the penile suspensory ligament [2]. The degloving incision allows complete inspection of the urethra and cavernosa [5]. Beginning with the deepest structures, namely the corpora cavernosa and corpus spongiosum, primary closure can be achieved in virtually all cases. The authors usually close injuries of the tunica albuginea in a transverse fashion to prevent narrowing of the corpora. With highly destructive bullet injuries, defects in the tunica albuginea may be so large as to preclude primary closure. In such instances, which are rare in civilian practice, off-the-shelf fascia, pericardium, or other collagen matrix type products may be helpful in achieving both hemostasis and a long-term functional outcome. For severe disruptions of the deep crural structures, plication maneuvers to exclude proximal crus may be feasible. Given the high likelihood of arterial injury with both blunt and penetrating disruption of the crura, arterial insufficiency and erectile dysfunction may occur regardless of techniques to repair the tunica albuginea.

Active bleeding, hematoma, and a defect in the fibers of the tunica albuginea all are characteristic of penile fractures and penetrating injuries to the corpus cavernosum (Fig. 2). The tunica albuginea

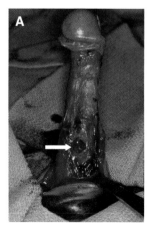
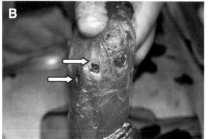

Fig. 2. Appearance of injuries to tunica albuginea. (*A*) Penile fracture exposed by degloving incision. Note clear disruption of tunica albuginea on lateral aspect of cavernosum extending toward corpus spongiosum (*arrow*). (*B*) Entry and exit wounds (*arrows*) to tunica albuginea from a low-velocity weapon.

is closed with interrupted slowly absorbable sutures. Although debridement and curettage may be indicated in cases presenting in a delayed fashion, most acute injuries do not require such maneuvers. Extensive irrigation, usually with a pulse lavage system and normal saline, is appropriate to remove any foreign body. In cases of penetrating impalement injuries or gunshot wounds, foreign material including clothing, missile fragments, or pieces of bone may enter into the deep structures of the penis and urinary tract [19]. These must be actively sought in such cases and removed (Fig. 3).

Injury to the glans penis presents a special challenge because of cosmetic concerns. Defects of glandular tissue do not preclude a good outcome. Debridement and trimming of skin edges to create a clean wound allow for closure of fairly large defects (Fig. 4A). Although the size of the glans may be reduced, its overall contour can usually be maintained. Circumcision injury in children often involves only the distal glans, which can be reattached as a free graft with acceptable results.

Most lacerations of the genital skin can be closed primarily (Fig. 5). The extensive and redundant blood supply of genital skin allows a greater flexibility and safety in wound closure than in other body areas. Simple uncontaminated bite injuries can be irrigated and closed primarily if appropriate antibiotics are administered, contamination is minimal, and the wound is closed within 6 to 12 hours [20]. Grossly contaminated bite injuries should be left open and allowed to granulate (Fig. 6). Similarly, most penetrating injuries to the penis and genitalia can be closed primarily as long as devitalized tissue is debrided, foreign material is removed, and appropriate antimicrobial coverage is given. Xeroform gauze and bulky fluffs loosely wrapped around the penis complete the

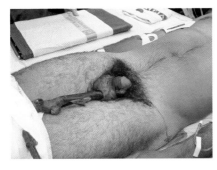

Fig. 3. Impalement of scrotum by stick. (Courtesy of Dr. Robert M. Sweet, Minneapolis, MN.)

dressing. Although some authors advocate pharmacologic treatment to prevent erections in the postoperative period, the authors have not found this approach to be necessary [21]. Local application of antibiotic ointments should be started once the dressings are taken down. Wound infections are uncommon after repair of penile injuries.

Injuries in uncircumcised patients present wound management issues. The redundant prepuce makes dressings more difficult; sometimes postoperative adhesions of the proximal shaft skin can lead to skin deformities. Nevertheless, the authors rarely perform simultaneous circumcision to preserve genital skin for possible future reconstruction.

A penile wound that requires special consideration is the circumferential full-thickness injury to the penile shaft skin (Fig. 7). Whether caused by an acute laceration, amputation, or constriction ring injury, the full-thickness loss of skin, subcutaneous tissues, and lymphatics can lead to permanent and disabling distal penile edema or skin sloughing. Simple lacerations of the base of the penis, even when circumferential, usually do not lead to complete interruption of lymphatic drainage, and should be closed primarily without immediate concern for distal penile edema. In contrast, after prolonged constriction ring placement with resulting ischemic necrosis, when full-thickness skin loss occurs there exists a much higher likelihood of subsequent lymph edema. Even in such circumstances, local care to the area of skin loss is the best initial management. If subsequent disabling edema occurs, the skin can be removed and replaced with a split-thickness skin graft. Fairly dramatic improvements have been observed with conservative therapy, however, and early aggressive debridement of viable skin is contraindicated. In cases of penile amputation, the best chance for skin survival is when complete microvascular reattachment including venous anastomosis is performed. When a simple cavernosal reanastomosis, without microvascular repair, is performed, skin loss is guaranteed.

Likewise, surgical management of burns, electrical injuries, and other skin injuries of the genitalia should be conservative [22]. The rich vascular supply may allow a greater degree of skin preservation than is expected in other areas of the genitalia. The authors' single institution experience with genital burns suggests that skin grafting for such injuries is a rare event (Fig. 8). Complete loss of genital skin usually implies a devastating burn from which patients may be unlikely

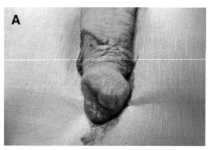
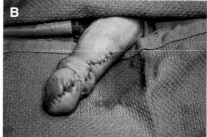

Fig. 4. Penile gunshot wound. (*A*) Injury to glans and superficial shaft of penis. (*B*) Final appearance of wounds after debridement of glans and primary skin closure with chromic suture.

to survive. In contrast, less than complete surface area burns of the genitalia have a remarkable capacity for recovery, and skin grafting is the exception rather than the rule [23].

Penile amputation requires precise management of urethral, cavernosal, neurovascular, and skin transsection in all but the most distal injuries. Simple urethral and tunica albugineal reapproximation of complete shaft amputation usually leads to survival and function of the organ, although skin loss is unavoidable and sensation of the glans and accompanying ejaculatory function is lost. Urethral stricture is also more common. Whenever possible, the authors advocate complete reattachment with microvascular and nerve reattachment. Critical issues include the quality of the amputated shaft and stump. With a clean cut, virtually no preparation is required (Fig. 9). If the penis has been avulsed or cut with a blunt instrument, or purposefully mutilated by the patient or the assailant, however, then reattachment may be problematic. Reattachment begins at the most ventral portion of the penis. Reapproximation starts with the tunica of the corpus spongiosum, the urethral epithelium over a catheter, followed by the ventral-most aspect of the tunica albuginea of the corpus cavernosum.

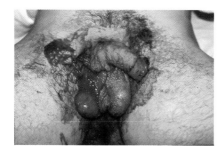

Fig. 5. Superficial skin lacerations caused by skill saw injury.

Reanastomosis of the deep arteries of the cavernosum usually is not required or easy. The authors only perform dorsal arterial reanastomosis. Once the tunica albuginea of the corpus cavernosum has been reapproximated, then the dorsal structures have brought in to proximity. The authors perform microvascular reanastomosis of one or both dorsal arteries, the dorsal nerves, and the deep dorsal vein. Failure to reanastomose the deep dorsal vein may lead to glans hyperemia and venous congestion of the shaft skin, which can compromise the success of the reattachment. Postoperatively, venous congestion is a major problem even with microvascular reattachment. The authors have found that the use of medical leeches is very helpful in reducing swelling and hematoma related to venous congestion and postoperative bleeding.

Injuries to the scrotum

Lacerations and avulsions of the scrotum not involving the testis may occur because of blunt trauma, machinery accidents, and stab wounds and occasional firearm injury. Complete avulsion of the scrotal skin is rare and is usually the result of power takeoff, auger, or devastating motor vehicle crashes involving widespread skin avulsion and degloving. Evaluation of the testis for potential rupture is mandatory and involves physical examination, scrotal ultrasonography, or direct exploration.

Scrotal skin lacerations can be closed primarily in the absence of gross infection or heavy contamination, and like penile skin, the scrotum is very resistant to ischemia and infection. Meticulous hemostasis is important because the scrotum accepts a large capacity of bleeding without tamponade. Layered closure of the deep fascia and skin, with a Penrose drain brought out dependently, limits postoperative hematoma (Fig. 10). Interrupted

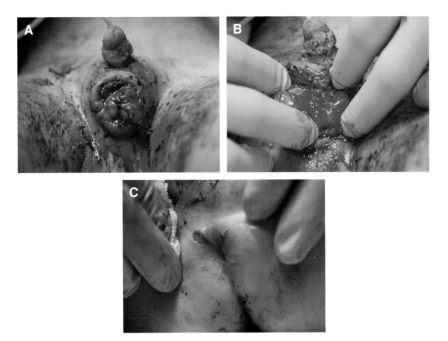

Fig. 6. Dog bite injury to male infant with gross contamination (*A*), intact tunica vaginalis (*B*), and perianal puncture wounds (*C*). Wounds were left open initially. Anoscopy revealed no other injuries.

closures reduce the likelihood of ischemia and may allow further drainage between the sutures. The authors always close the deep layer with an absorbable suture. Skin closures vary; usually, absorbable monofilament, such chromic or synthetic substitutes, works well. In some cases with challenging wound characteristics, nonabsorbable sutures, such as nylon, may be preferable. Xeroform gauze or other antibacterial dressings and ointments should be placed on the incisions, and the scrotum should be surrounded with fluffed gauze and a supporting meshed panty.

Complete scrotal avulsion is a devastating injury. It may be possible to preserve avulsed skin sheared off in a motor vehicle crash, and prepare it for immediate full- or split-thickness skin grafting. Machinery injuries with rotating mechanisms may damage the intrinsic microvasculature of the skin and make it unsuitable for grafting. In the absence of devastating burns or massive skin injuries, the authors do not advocate immediate grafting but rather favor an interval of local care and dressing changes with saline-soaked gauze. This ensures that contamination is removed

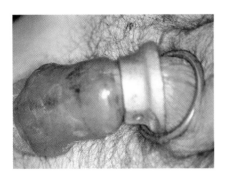

Fig. 7. Constriction device with distal edema and duskiness.

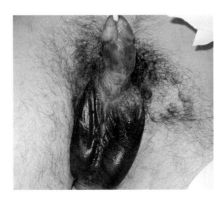

Fig. 8. Caustic chemical burn to the scrotum and penis. (Courtesy of Dr. Robert M. Sweet, Minneapolis, MN.)

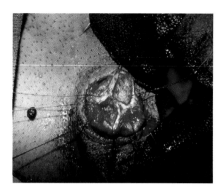

Fig. 9. Appearance of penile stump after amputation. Note well-delineated cavernosal anatomy that allowed replantation. (Courtesy of Dr. Jack W. McAninch, San Francisco, CA.)

and allows the bed to granulate, after which very successful results can be obtained with split-thickness skin grafts obtained from thigh donor sites [24]. Testicular transplantation into subcutaneous thigh pouches is not frequently required for traumatic injuries to the scrotum. It can be a temporizing or permanent measure, however, dependent on patient age, sexual function, and overall prioritization of trauma injuries.

Injuries to the female genitalia

Female genital injuries are especially morbid given their mechanisms involving severe pelvic fractures or sexual assault and interpersonal violence. Many vulvar lacerations are the result of sports-related straddle-type injuries [25–28]. Genital trauma, however, is reported in 20% to 53% of sexual assault victims [1,29]. Such a history must be sought. If elicited, appropriate support

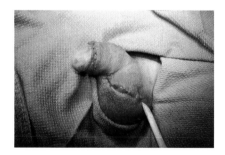

Fig. 10. Primary closure of penile and scrotal lacerations (same patient as in Fig. 5) with dependent drainage of wounds.

services and police involvement must be secured [30]. Furthermore, informed consent for the rest of the patient assessment should be obtained if a history of sexual assault has been verified. Required assessment includes history, physical examination, and collection of laboratory and forensic specimens as outlined by the American College of Obstetrics and Gynecologists [31].

Table 3 shows the characteristics of injuries to the vagina and vulva, and corresponding AIS scores. Regardless of the mechanism, all female patients with external genital injuries should be suspected of having injury to the internal female organs and the lower urinary tract and urethra. Many female urethral injuries are associated with vaginal bleeding, and the possibility of pelvic fracture or impalement injury should prompt especially diligent evaluation [32]. This includes cystourethrography, proctoscopy, and laparotomy as indicated. The failure to identify associated urinary tract and gastrointestinal injuries in the face of vaginal trauma may lead to abscess formation, sepsis, and death.

Table 3
AAST organ injury scale for female genital injury

Injured structure	AAST grade	Characteristics of injury	AIS-90 score
Vagina	I	Contusion or hematoma	1
	II	Superficial laceration (mucosa only)	1
	III	Deep laceration (into fat or muscle)	2
	IV	Complex laceration (into cervix or peritoneum)	3
	V	Injury to adjacent organs (anus, rectum, urethra, bladder)	3
Vulva	I	Contusion or hematoma	1
	II	Superficial laceration (skin only)	1
	III	Deep laceration (into fat or muscle)	2
	IV	Avulsion (skin, fat, or muscle)	3
	V	Injury to adjacent organs (anus, rectum, urethra, bladder)	3

Abbreviations: AAST, American Association for the Surgery of Trauma; AIS, Abbreviated Injury Scale.

Perineal and vulvar lacerations can usually be managed in the emergency department. Large hematomas should be incised and drained, with ligation of any bleeding vessels. As with the male genital skin, closure with interruptive absorbable sutures is standard. Drains can be used if there is a large cavity, if hemostasis is suboptimal, or if there is suspected contamination [27].

Internal lacerations to the vagina and cervix can be closed in the emergency department as long as there is not severe bleeding. Large lacerations associated with bleeding and hematoma require speculum examination under anesthesia to completely assess and repair the injuries. Vaginal lacerations are closed with continuous absorbable sutures, and vaginal packing is critical for hemostasis.

Complex vaginal and perineal lacerations, associated with pelvic fracture, rectal injury, or other adverse features require a more systematic approach. Evaluation under anesthesia is mandatory including speculum examination, cystoscopy or cystography, and rigid proctoscopy. Diversion of the fecal stream is rarely indicated unless perineal injuries extensively involve the rectum, anus, or external sphincter. Bladder ruptures should be repaired if associated vaginal lacerations are present, to prevent deep pelvic infection and abscess or formation of vesicovaginal fistulae.

Summary

Genital anatomy has evolved to maximize protection of reproductive function from blunt trauma. When weapons, excessive bending, or shear forces exceed the threshold for deformation, however, rupture and bleeding are inevitable. Important contextual issues include potential criminal violence, associated pelvic organ injury, and importance of preserved function and cosmesis. The ultimate goal of reconstructive surgery is to preserve genitalia with normal function and appearance. Prompt operative management of deep injuries to the penis and vagina controls bleeding and reduces the likelihood of later sexual dysfunction. Primary closure of most wounds including uncomplicated bites and penetrating injuries is possible with appropriate antibiotic administration. Delayed closure and skin grafting can salvage wounds complicated by a delay in diagnosis, avulsion, contamination, or secondary necrotizing infection. Finally, complete amputation is best treated at tertiary centers that can perform microvascular complete reattachment.

References

[1] Sugar NF, Fine DN, Eckert LO. Physical injury after sexual assault: findings of a large case series. Am J Obstet Gynecol 2004;190:71–6.

[2] Morey AF, Metro MJ, Carney KJ, et al. Consensus on genitourinary trauma: external genitalia. BJU Int 2004;94:507–15.

[3] Mohr AM, Pham AM, Lavery RF, et al. Management of trauma to the male external genitalia: the usefulness of American Association for the Surgery of Trauma organ injury scales. J Urol 2003;170 (6 Pt 1):2311–5.

[4] Thompson IM, Flaherty SF, Morey AF. Battlefield urologic injuries: the Gulf War experience. J Am Coll Surg 1998;187:139–41.

[5] Mydlo J. Blunt and penetrating trauma to the penis. In: Wessells H, McAninch JM, editors. Urological emergencies: a practical guide, vol 1. 1st edition. Totowa: Humana; 2005. p. 95–112.

[6] Penson DF, Seftel AD, Krane RJ, et al. The hemodynamic pathophysiology of impotence following blunt trauma to the erect penis. J Urol 1992;148:1171–80.

[7] Zargooshi J. Penile fracture in Kermanshah, Iran: report of 172 cases. J Urol 2000;164:364–6.

[8] Adigun IA, Kuranga SA, Abdulrahman LO. Grinding machine: friend or foe. West Afr J Med 2002;21: 338–40.

[9] Jezior JR, Brady JD, Schlossberg SM. Management of penile amputation injuries. World J Surg 2001;25: 1602–9.

[10] Aboseif SGR, McAninch JW. Genital self-mutilation. J Urol 1993;150:1143.

[11] Armenakas NA, McAninch JW, Lue TF, et al. Posttraumatic impotence: magnetic resonance imaging and duplex ultrasound in diagnosis and management. J Urol 1993;149(5 Pt 2):1272–5.

[12] Eke N. Urological complications of coitus. BJU Int 2002;89:273–7.

[13] Cline KJ, Mata JA, Venable DD, et al. Penetrating trauma to the male external genitalia. Journal of Trauma-Injury Infection & Critical Care 1998;44: 492–4.

[14] Michielsen D, Neetens C, Lafaire C, et al. Burns to the genitalia and perineum. J Urol 1998;159:418.

[15] Jabren GW, Hellstrom WJG. Trauma to the external genitalia. In: Wessells H, McAninch JM, editors. Urological emergencies: a practical guide. Totowa: Humana; 2005. p. 71–93.

[16] Talan DACD, Abrahamian FM, Moran GJ, et al. Bacteriologic analysis of infected dog and cat bites. N Engl J Med 1999;340:85.

[17] Wolf JS, McAninch JW. Human bites to the penis. J Urol 1992;147:1265.

[18] Gross H. The role of cavernosography in acute fracture of the penis. Radiology 1982;144:787.

[19] Poulton TL, Wessells H. Delayed presentation of an intravesical foreign body 6 years after impalement injury. J Urol 2003;169:1792.

[20] Fleisher GR. The management of bite wounds. N Engl J Med 1999;340:138.

[21] Mydlo JH, Harris CF, Brown JG. Blunt, penetrating and ischemic injuries to the penis. J Urol 2002;168 (4 Pt 1):1433–5.

[22] McAninch JW. Management of genital skin loss. Urol Clin North Am 1989;16:387–97.

[23] Peck BM, Grube BJ, Heimbach DM. The management of burns to the perineum and genitals. J Burn Care Rehabil 1990;11:54.

[24] Wessells H. Genital skin loss: unified reconstructive approach to a heterogeneous entity. World J Urol 1999;17:107–14.

[25] Haefner HK, Andersen HF, Johnson MP. Vaginal laceration following a jet-ski accident. Obstet Gynecol 1991;78(5 Pt 2):986–8.

[26] Mandell J, Cromie WJ, Caldamone AA. Sports-related genitourinary injuries in children. Clin Sports Med 1982;1:483–93.

[27] Knudson MM, Crombleholme WR. Female genital trauma and sexual assault. In: Blaidsell FW, Trunkey DD, editors. Abdominal trauma. New York: Thieme Medical Publishers; 1993. p. 311–23.

[28] Merrit D. Evaluating and managing acute genital trauma in premenarchal girls. J Pediatr Adolesc Gynecol 1999;12:237–8.

[29] Riggs N, Houry D, Long G, et al. Analysis of 1,076 cases of sexual assault. Ann Emerg Med 2000;35: 358–62.

[30] Bottomley CP, Sadler T, Welch J. Integrated clinical service for sexual assault victims in a genitourinary setting. Sex Transm Infect 1999;75:116–9.

[31] American College of Obstetricians and Gynecologists (ACOG). Sexual Assault. ACOG Educ Bull 1997 Nov;(242):1–7.

[32] Niemi TA, Norton LW. Vaginal injuries in patients with pelvic fracture. J Trauma 1985;25:547–51.

ELSEVIER
SAUNDERS

Urol Clin N Am 33 (2006) 127–131

UROLOGIC
CLINICS
of North America

Index

Note: Page numbers of article titles are in **boldface** type.

0094-0143/06/$ - see front matter © 2006 Elsevier Inc. All rights reserved.
doi:10.1016/S0094-0143(06)00010-3

urologic.theclinics.com

Changing Your Address?

Make sure your subscription changes too! When you notify us of your new address, you can help make our job easier by including an exact copy of your Clinics label number with your old address (see illustration below.) This number identifies you to our computer system and will speed the processing of your address change. Please be sure this label number accompanies your old address and your corrected address—you can send an old Clinics label with your number on it or just copy it exactly and send it to the address listed below.

We appreciate your help in our attempt to give you continuous coverage. Thank you.

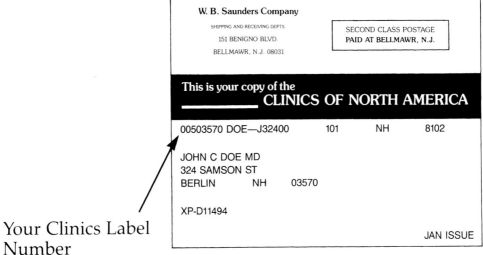

Your Clinics Label Number
Copy it exactly or send your label along with your address to:
W.B. Saunders Company, Customer Service
Orlando, FL 32887-4800
Call Toll Free 1-800-654-2452

Please allow four to six weeks for delivery of new subscriptions and for processing address changes.